200
BRAIDS
to twist, knot,
loop, or weave

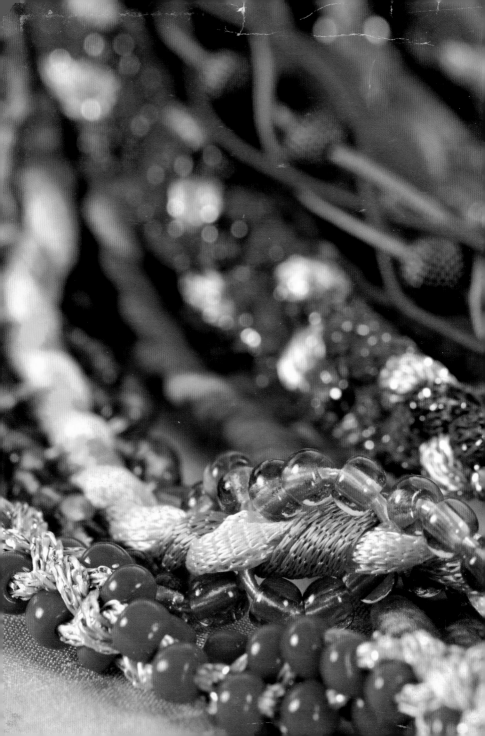

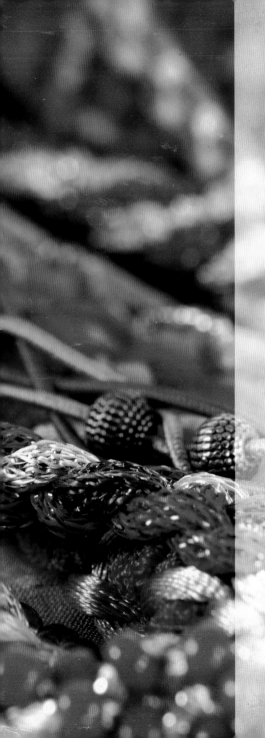

200
BRAIDS
to twist, knot,
loop, or weave

Jacqui Carey

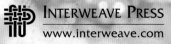
INTERWEAVE PRESS
www.interweave.com

A QUARTO BOOK

Copyright © 2007 Quarto Inc.

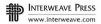
INTERWEAVE PRESS
www.interweave.com

Published in North America by
Interweave Press LLC
201 East Fourth Street
Loveland, CO 80537-5655
www.interweave.com
All rights reserved.

Conceived, designed, and produced by
Quarto Publishing plc
The Old Brewery
6 Blundell Street
London N7 9BH

QUA.BRBI

Library of Congress Cataloging-in-Publication Data
Carey, Jacqui.
200 braids to twist, knot, loop, or weave / Jacqui Carey,
author.
p. cm.
Includes index.
ISBN 10: 1–59668–018–0
ISBN 13: 978–1–59668–018–0
1. Braid. 2. Hand weaving. I. Title. II. Title: Two hundred
braids to twist, knot, loop, or weave.
TT848.C28 2007
746.1'4041--dc22

Senior editor: Liz Pasfield
Art editor: Natasha Montgomery
Copy editor: Sue Richardson
Designers: John Thompson, Michelle Stamp, Jill Mumford
Assistant art director: Penny Cobb
Photographers: Philip Wilkins, Karl Adamson
Illustrator: Kuo Kang Chen
Picture research: Claudia Tate

Art director: Moira Clinch
Publisher: Paul Carslake

Color separation by Modern Age Repro House Ltd,
Hong Kong
Printed in China by Midas Printing International Ltd

10 9 8 7 6 5 4 3 2 1

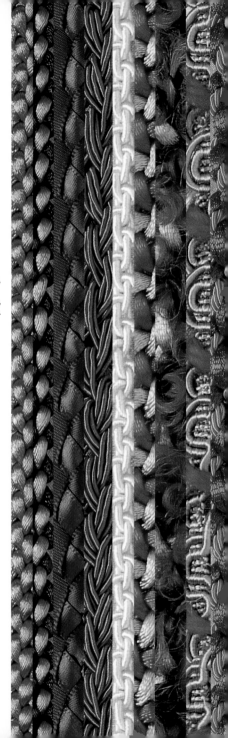

CONTENTS

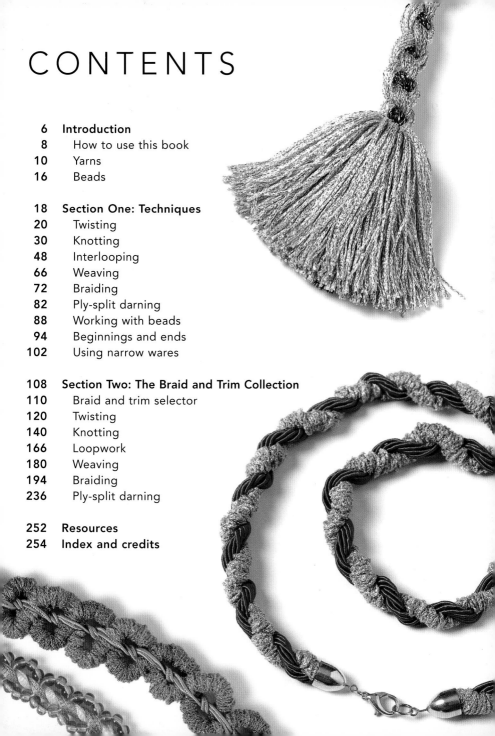

Introduction

Everyone needs a braid at some time in their life—whether to finish off a beautifully handcrafted project or just to tie things together. Braiding is an ancient technique that has been utilized for its strength and flexibility, as well as its beauty. Braids are everywhere in our modern lives but are rarely noticed; from the laces on our shoes to the hoses in our cars. However, finding the perfect trim for a particular project is often impossible unless it is handmade especially for the purpose.

This book provides you with a whole range of trim possibilities that are all easy and require little or no equipment. This means that anyone can dip in and find a solution to their needs. You don't need to be dedicated to this subject to use or need this book. You don't need to be a trimmings or narrow wares expert to create the perfect finishing touch for your project. These narrow wares can complement so many other techniques— not just textile ones.

The word braid means different things to different people, though to be specific it has been defined as "oblique interlacing." This book contains different methods of producing narrow wares— twisting, knotting, interlooping, weaving, braiding, and ply-split darning. Each of these methods is explained, with step-by-step photos. Samples of each method are detailed showing a range of possibilities and patterns to be explored.

Jacqui Carey

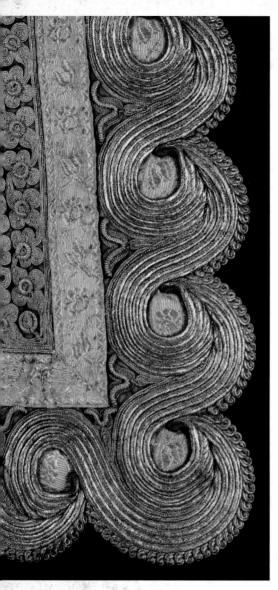

Above: A detail of the edging of a mid-nineteenth century Albanian embroidered coat showing braids.
Right: A detail of a Englishman's jacket from the early seventeenth century, showing knotted narrow wares couched down.

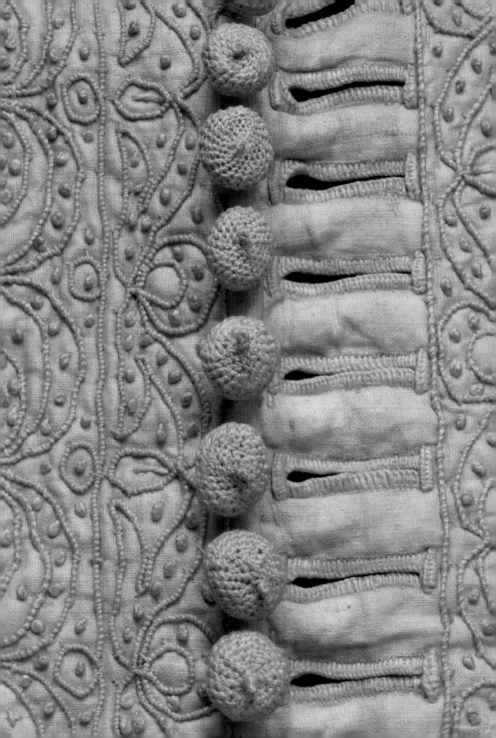

How to use this book

The book is divided into two parts. To begin with you will find useful information on yarns and beads and all of the core techniques required to make the braids shown in the book. The Braid and Trim Collection is divided into smaller sections showing examples of braids that have been twisted, knotted, looped, woven, braided, or ply-split.

WORKING PRACTICE

In this section of the book you'll find useful information on yarns and beads that can be used to create the beautiful braids in this book. Moving onto techiques, you will find easy-to-follow steps showing all of the techniques used in the book. Start to practice the key moves and soon you'll be creating your own variations.

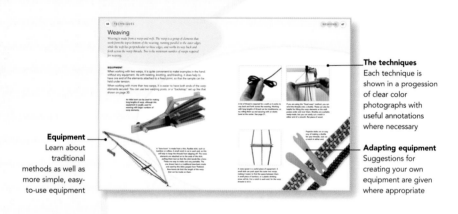

Equipment
Learn about traditional methods as well as more simple, easy-to-use equipment

The techniques
Each technique is shown in a progression of clear color photographs with useful annotations where necessary

Adapting equipment
Suggestions for creating your own equipment are given where appropriate

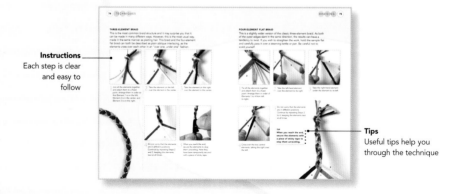

Instructions
Each step is clear and easy to follow

Tips
Useful tips help you through the technique

THE BRAID AND TRIM COLLECTION

A beautiful reference chapter that shows examples of narrow wares created from all of the techniques in the book. You can also use the selector on pages 110–119 to quickly find a design that appeals to you.

Diagram
A useful diagram reminds you of the technique

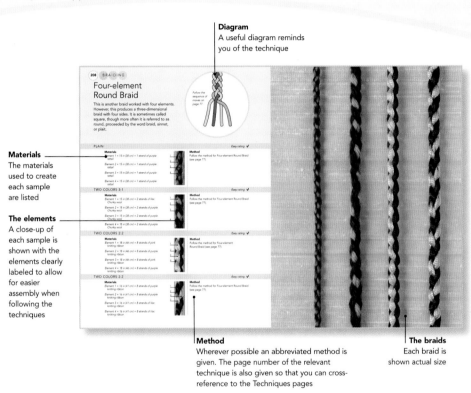

Materials
The materials used to create each sample are listed

The elements
A close-up of each sample is shown with the elements clearly labeled to allow for easier assembly when following the techniques

Method
Wherever possible an abbreviated method is given. The page number of the relevant technique is also given so that you can cross-reference to the Techniques pages

The braids
Each braid is shown actual size

TAKE-UP RATES

With each braid you will see the length of the element required to make a 12 in. (30 cm) sample. The take-up will change depending on the yarn size and elasticity, the nature of the working method used, as well as the tension added by the individual worker. Take-up is not an exact science, so the lengths given in the book are only a guide. Even if all the ingredients are the same, the take-up rate will vary from person to person. You will often find that if you repeat the same sample several times over, the chances are that the take-up will vary between them. If you have a particular project in mind, it is better to allow too much than too little. It is easier to cut something down to size than to try to join strands together.

Yarns

Narrow wares can be made from any fiber or thread. Each different texture will produce a different result, so you can get just the effect you are after. Generally, smooth shiny threads give more precise results, while fluffier threads give softer, fuzzier effects. You can try mixing different fibers together to achieve some stunning combinations, though be aware that the elasticity of different yarns can affect the result.

The length of yarn you will need for each project will vary depending on what is known as "take-up," (see page 9 for more information).

COTTON AND SYNTHETIC YARNS

There is a wide selection available of cotton and synthetic yarns that are suitable for creating the braids in this book.

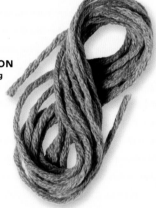

CALMER COTTON

This is a 2-ply yarn with each ply consisting of a knitted chain. It is a mix of cotton and acrylic that has a soft appearance and gives a tactile result.

DOUBLE TOP COTTON

This is a 4-ply cotton yarn that gives a soft and chunky result. This is a versatile yarn with a good weight for creating braids.

GLITTER VISCOSE

This yarn is a mix of viscose and Lurex of knitted construction. The glint of metallic adds a subtle sparkle to braids without making them too glittery.

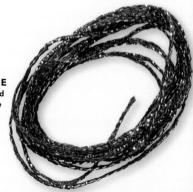

KNITTING RIBBON

This yarn is made from a viscose fiber constructed into hollow tubular knitting. It is a very flexible and versatile yarn and provides a smooth and shiny result.

PEARL COTTON

A tightly spun 2-ply cotton yarn that is available in several weights. For the construction of some of the braids in this book both No. 5 (a medium weight) and No. 8 (a slightly finer weight) have been used. Both provide a firm and slightly glossy result.

RUCHED KNITTING RIBBON

This is the knitting ribbon shown above but with an inner core added into the center of the hollow tube. The inner core can be any yarn, for example, two lengths of pearl cotton. The knitting ribbon can then be ruched along the core thread to create a ruched, shiny effect. This can be done by hand.

PRISM VISCOSE

This is a high-luster 2-ply viscose. It is a strong and crisp fiber giving precise results. However, it can be rather slippery to work with.

SPECIALTY YARNS

It can also be interesting to add specialty wools and knitting yarns to your braids.

BALMORAL
BOUCLÉ

This is a looped yarn of soft wool, made with a black ply and loosely spun colored loops. This yarn gives a fuzzy and textured result.

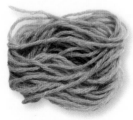

RIBBON TWIST

This is a wool yarn teamed with an acrylic knitted ribbon and plied together with a fine black polymide thread. It provides a chunky soft result with a subtle flash of constrasting color and texture.

TWEED YARN

This tweed-effect yarn is made from 70% silk and 30% cotton. The result is a noile that is textured to look at and to feel.

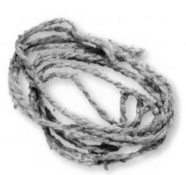

KID CLASSIC WOOL

A 4-ply yarn spun from lambswool and kid mohair. It is a soft and fuzzy yarn with a subtle glint of sheen.

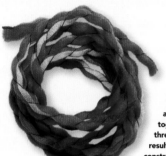

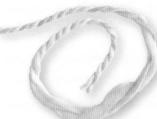

BABY SOFT WOOL

This is a 2-ply wool with a subtle slub that when used in creating braids gives varied thicknesses.

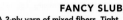

FANCY SLUB

A 2-ply yarn of mixed fibers. Tight slubs of different colors give the yarn an exciting texture and varied thicknesses.

CHUNKY WOOL

This yarn is a thick 4-ply wool. It is a robust yarn that doesn't give too much fuzziness in the finished results.

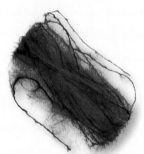

KIDSILK HAZE

A fine yarn made up of 70% kid mohair and 30% silk giving a soft and very fuzzy result.

TINSEL YARN

This is a Lurex and viscose chenille-style yarn that gives a furry effect to braids with an added sparkle.

OTHER YARNS AND PREMADE NARROW WARES

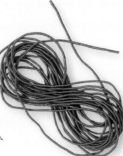

GIMP

Gimp is a thick, smooth yarn made from viscose wrapped around a cotton core. This yarn gives braids a crisp and clean line.

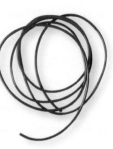

PLASTIC TUBING

This thick and smooth material is hollow. It is not as flexible as a fiber yarn.

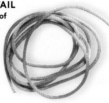

RATTAIL

This is a thick, smooth yarn of tightly interworked viscose fibers. Rattail is a thicker and more flexible yarn than gimp.

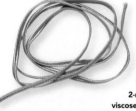

RUSSIA BRAID

This is a machine-made 2-ridge braid created by viscose over a cotton core. This is a firm but flexible yarn.

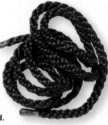

CREPE CORD

A thick 3-ply viscose cord. Each ply is made from a 2-ply-cord. A finer version of crepe cord is called lacing cord.

RIBBON

Flat woven ribbons are available in many different widths and colors. They can be worked flat, folded, or scrunched up to give different effects.

JAPANESE BRAID

This silk braid is made by machine. It has a 4-ridge square shape with a stiff tension that means that it acts with a wirelike firmness when being used to create narrow wares.

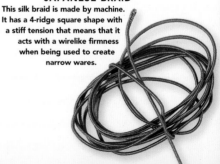

MAKING AN ELEMENT

The yarns can be used as single strands, but many samples require several strands to be worked together to make a single element. You can just gather together the required number, but if you want the strands to be even, then it is worth preparing the elements in the following manner. This example shows you how to prepare an element of eight strands of cotton.

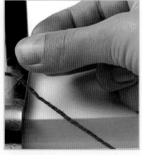

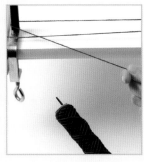

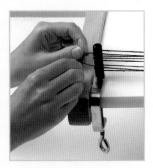

1 Hold, tape, or tie one end of the strand to one winding post.

2 Wind the strand around the posts, counting each time you arrive at a post (one for each required strand), here 2 strands have been prepared and the third is starting.

3 Continue winding until you have the required number of strands prepared. Here a total of 8 strands have been made. Knot the start and finish of the strand. The strands between the posts are the required amount for one element. You can take them off the posts and continue with your chosen method. If you need more than one element, you can prepare them singly, as shown above, or you can prepare them all together.

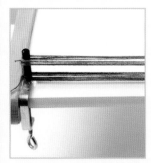

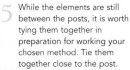

5 While the elements are still between the posts, it is worth tying them together in preparation for working your chosen method. Tie them together close to the post.

4 Here, 8 strands of dark green cotton have been wound around the post and knotted together. They have been pushed low down the posts. Next, 8 strands of light green cotton have been wound around the posts and knotted. There are now two elements-worth of cotton between the posts.

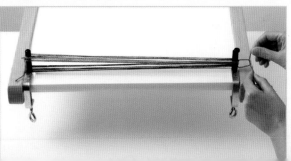

Beads

There are many different types of beads available today. They come in a whole range of shapes, sizes, and materials. The wide choice of colors means that it is easy to find beads to coordinate with your yarns. The variety of beads makes for a wonderful choice, but variation can be an issue when trying to identify a matching bead. For example, the small glass beads known as seed, or rocaille beads are sold in sizes such as 11°, 10°, 8 °, and 6°. This should be helpful to find the right size bead for a project (the larger the number, the smaller the bead). However, even if the beads are labeled as the same size, you will find variations between different suppliers. There are also discrepancies in the size of the bead holes. These often vary, even within the same batch. So be prepared to find a few that will not fit over the needle. The beads here are shown actual size with a single enlarged bead shown next to each group.

SEED BEADS

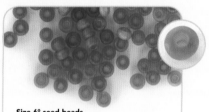

Size 6° seed beads
Seed beads usually come from Japan or the Czech Republic, although there are several other countries that produce them. The Japanese beads tend to be slightly larger and have a larger hole than the Czech beads.

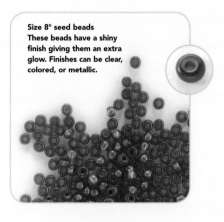

Size 8° seed beads
These beads have a shiny finish giving them an extra glow. Finishes can be clear, colored, or metallic.

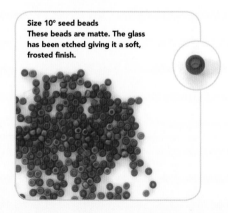

Size 10° seed beads
These beads are matte. The glass has been etched giving it a soft, frosted finish.

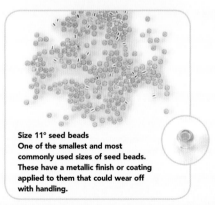

Size 11° seed beads
One of the smallest and most commonly used sizes of seed beads. These have a metallic finish or coating applied to them that could wear off with handling.

LARGER BEADS

Larger bead types can also be used to add embellishment and interest to your braids.

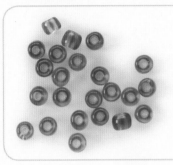

4mm glass beads
Plain round glass beads come in a range of sizes and colors and are an easy and useful way of embellishing your braids.

Pony beads
These beads are fairly large—around ¼ in. (1 cm) in size—and donut shaped. They are reasonably regular in size and are useful for producing large features where plenty of thread can go through the hole in the bead.

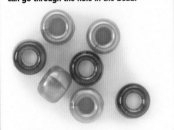

Chip beads
Chip beads are small, random-shaped pieces of semiprecious stones that have been polished and pierced. They will give a shiny but irregular texture to your work.

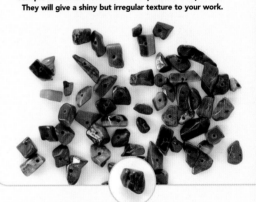

Size 2 beads
A smaller-size glass bead with an interesting color-lined hole. Sometimes in glass beads this can be a separate layer of glass, or it can be a fine layer of paint applied to the inside of the bead.

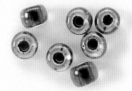

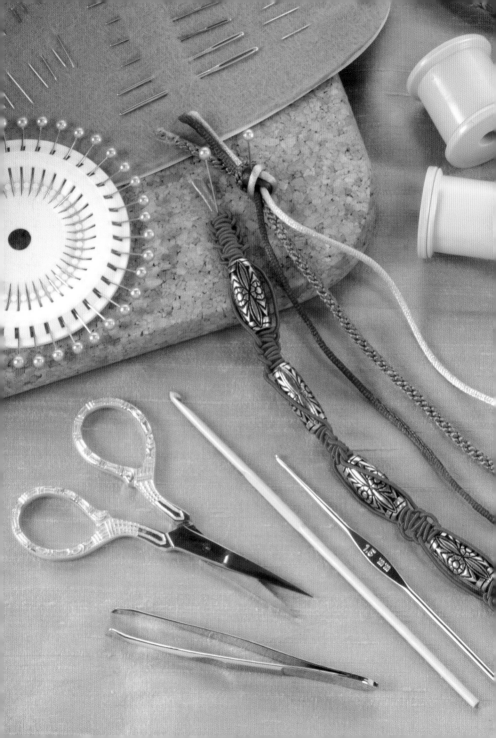

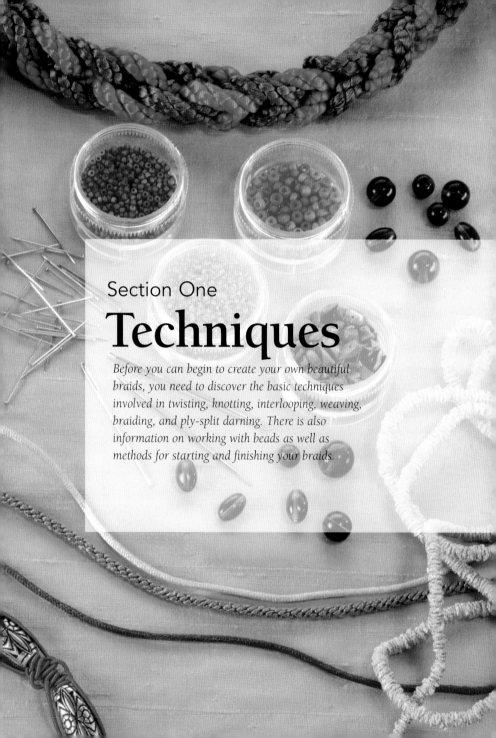

Section One

Techniques

Before you can begin to create your own beautiful braids, you need to discover the basic techniques involved in twisting, knotting, interlooping, weaving, braiding, and ply-split darning. There is also information on working with beads as well as methods for starting and finishing your braids.

Twisting

Twisting elements together is one of the oldest and most basic textile techniques. The process has many names such as "throwing," "plying," "doubling," or "cordspinning," depending on the context and the materials used. Different twisting methods can be found all over the world.

EQUIPMENT

You can work without equipment—for example, the ends of the elements can be clamped with the foot while the other ends are rolled between the hands. Rolling the elements between the hand and thigh is another possibility. However, it is much easier to tie the ends of the elements to a fixed point such as a warping post, coat hook, or door handle. The other ends can then be twisted, either with the hands or with the aid of equipment. Whatever you use, make sure that the ends of the elements remain secure at all times. Twisted cords are simply held together by the opposing twist in the thread, and they will unravel at the slightest opportunity. If you are using equipment, you will need to make sure that the end of the elements are looped so that the equipment can be inserted through the loop. You can always knot the threads together to make a loop. If you don't have access to equipment, a hand drill with a cup hook in the drill bit is also efficient.

There are many tools that have been specially designed for making cords. Here a special cord winder is being used to twist the threads. The threads are knotted to form a loop that goes over the hook.

TIP
Have a supply of cut lengths of sticky tape ready for use. These can be used to secure the twist temporarily, until a more permanent finish can be made.

TIP
The more twist you add to the elements the firmer the resulting cord will be.

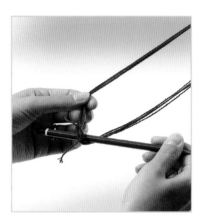

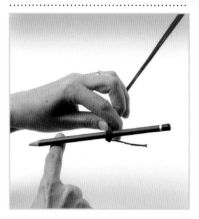

1 Something as simple as a pencil can speed up the winding process. Use it to help with the twisting by placing it into the end of the loops.

2 Gently pinch the threads with your left hand, just above the pencil. Use the tip of your right index finger to twirl the pencil as if it was an airplane propeller.

TWIST DIRECTION

The twist can be created in either direction. The twists take their names from the diagonal slants of the corresponding letters.

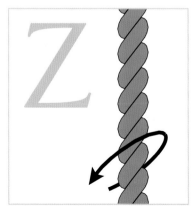

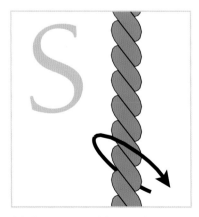

If the first twist is to the right (clockwise), then the final result will be a Z-twist cord.

If the first twist is to the left (counterclockwise), then the final result will be an S-twist cord.

TWO-PLY CORD

In theory, any number of elements could be used to make a twisted cord. However, the usual range is between two and four. Two-ply is made from two elements that are twisted together. The following instructions are for a Z-twist cord. If you wish to make an S-twist cord, then you must reverse all of the twist directions.

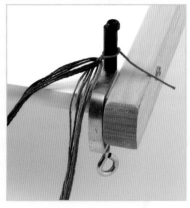

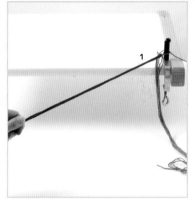

1 Tie the start of both elements together and attach them to a fixed point. Here they are joined to a warping post with a piece of spare thread.

2 Hold the far end of Element 1 and pull it taut away from the post.

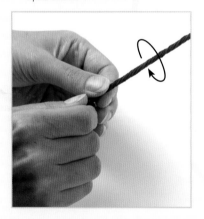

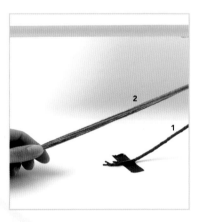

3 Twist Element 1 in a clockwise direction.

4 When Element 1 is fully twisted, secure it so that it is taut away from the post (here it has been secured to the table with sticky tape). Now take Element 2 and hold it taut away from the post. Note that it is longer than the other, twisted element.

TIP
Try to put the same amount of twist into both elements.

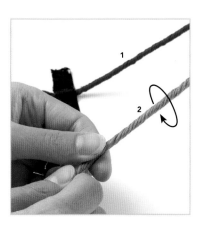

5 Twist Element 2 in a clockwise direction.

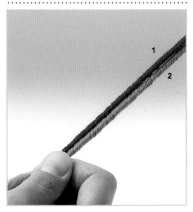

6 When Element 2 is fully twisted, bring the ends of both elements together. Make sure they are still taut away from the post.

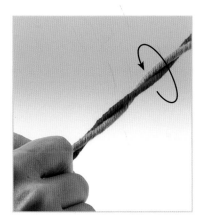

7 Twist the two elements together in a counterclockwise direction.

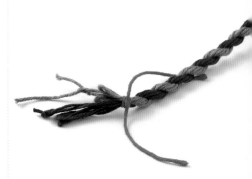

8 Secure the ends to stop them unraveling. This can be a temporary tie, such as the piece of spare thread shown here.

CABLING WITH ONE CORD

When a cord is retwisted it is known as "cabling." One or both elements of a two-ply cord can be a premade cord, and this gives an interesting texture to the finished result. Here a single cord is premade, then joined to more strands and retwisted to produce a textured cord. It is important to make sure that the premade cord is retwisted in the correct direction, so that the twist is tightened rather than loosened. The instructions use a Z-twist cord as one of the elements. If you wish to use an S-twist cord, don't forget to reverse all the twist directions.

1 Element 1 is a Z-twist, two-ply cord (see page 21). Join the start of the cord to the start of Element 2, tying them together with some spare thread.

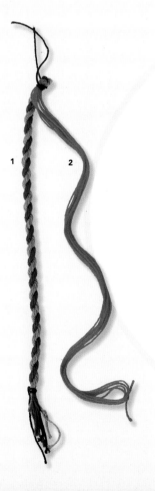

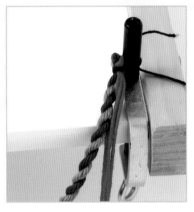

2 Attach the joined elements to a fixed point. Here they are joined to a warping post with a piece of spare thread.

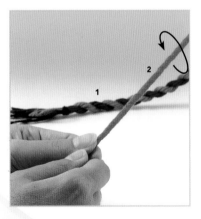

3 Hold the far end of Element 2 and pull it taut away from the post. Twist Element 2 in a counterclockwise direction. When Element 2 is fully twisted, secure it so that it is taut away from the post.

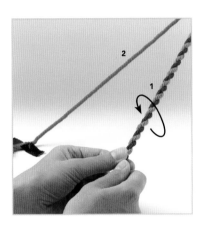

4   Now take Element 1 (the premade cord) and hold it taut away from the post. Twist Element 1 in a counterclockwise direction.

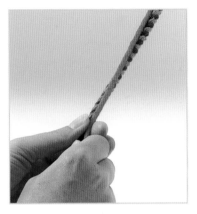

5   When Element 1 is fully twisted, bring the ends of both Element 2 and Element 1 together. Make sure they are still taut away from the post.

6   Twist Element 1 and Element 2 together in a clockwise direction. Secure the ends to stop them unraveling. Here they have been temporarily secured with some sticky tape.

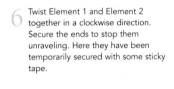

CABLING WITH TWO CORDS

Here both of the elements are premade cords. It is important that they are both made so that they twist in the same direction. You cannot cable a Z-twist and an S-twist cord together.

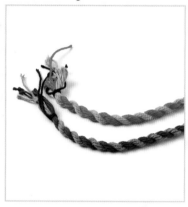

1 Take two Z-twist, two-ply cords (see page 21) and join the starts together.

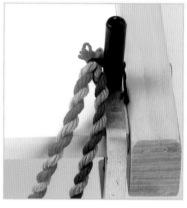

2 Attach the starts to a fixed point. Here they are tied to a warping post.

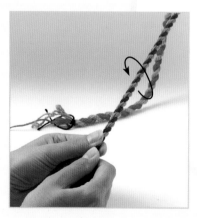

3 Hold the far end of one of the cords and pull it taut away from the post. Twist it in a counterclockwise direction.

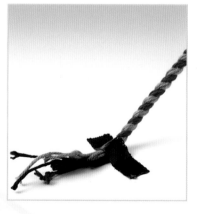

4 When it is fully twisted, secure it so that it is taut away from the post. Here it has been secured to the table with sticky tape.

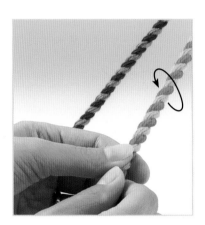

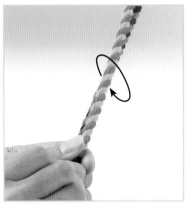

5   Now take the other cord and hold it taut away from the post. Twist it in a counterclockwise direction.

6   When it is fully twisted, bring the ends of both elements together. Make sure they are still taut away from the post. Twist them together in a clockwise direction.

7   Secure the ends to stop them unraveling. Here they have been temporarily secured with some sticky tape.

THREE-PLY CORD

When three elements are used to create a cord, it is known as three-ply. A little care is needed to keep the plies in the correct order. Ideally, they should be twisted together in an orderly fashion. However, if you are working alone and do not have special equipment, this can be a little tricky, but do not worry as the plies can be maneuvered after the cord is finished. The following instructions produce a Z-twist cord. If you wish to make an S-twist cord, then you must reverse all of the twist directions.

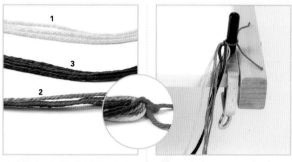

1 Tie the starts of Element 1, Element 2, and Element 3 together.

2 Attach the starts to a fixed point. Here they have been tied to a warping post with some spare thread.

3 Hold the far end of Element 1 and pull it taut away from the post. Twist it in a clockwise direction.

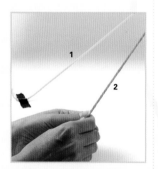

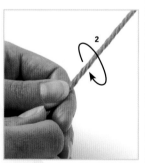

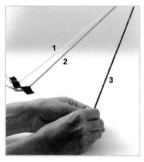

4 When Element 1 is fully twisted, secure it so that it is taut away from the post (here it has been secured to the table with sticky tape). Now take Element 2 and hold it taut away from the post.

5 Twist Element 2 in a clockwise direction.

6 When Element 2 is fully twisted, secure it so that it is taut away from the post. Now take Element 3 and hold it taut away from the post.

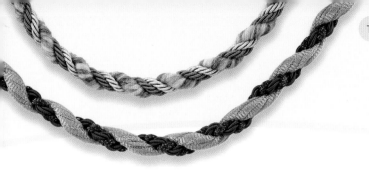

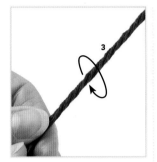

7 Twist Element 3 in a clockwise direction.

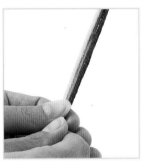

8 When Element 3 is fully twisted, bring the ends of all of the elements together. Make sure they are still taut away from the post.

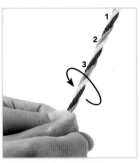

9 Twist the three elements together in a counterclockwise direction.

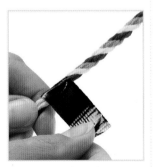

10 Secure the ends to stop them unraveling. Here they have been temporarily secured with some sticky tape.

TIP
Use chopsticks or knitting needles to help settle the plies out.

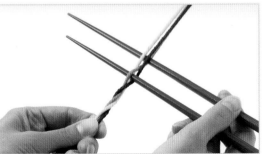

Before you finally twist the three plies together, insert a chopstick through the three plies, close to the end near your hand. Take it over, under, and over the plies. Insert the other chopstick, but take this under, over, and under. As you add the final twist, gradually ease the chopsticks toward the fixed point.

Knotting

Broadly speaking, knotting is a technique where elements make loops, and the ends of the elements are then taken through these loops and tightened. Although most knots are functional, they can also be used to create decorative narrow wares, some of which are well known, such as "macramé," "boondoggle," and "friendship bracelets."

EQUIPMENT

You don't need any equipment to do knotting, but sometimes you may find that it is helpful to tie or pin down some of the threads. This helps with the tensioning, and means you can keep your hands free to work the other threads. Some people like to work on a pin board so that all the threads can lie flat on a surface. Usually the best method is to attach the start of the work to a fixed point. You can tie your threads onto a post, chair back, or door handle—but be careful that the door is not suddenly opened! You can even tie the threads to your foot. When the start is secured, you can then pull the work away from the post so that the threads can be held taut. Occasionally some of the elements need to be held taut at all times. If this is the case, you can tie both ends of the elements. This will keep the tension constant, as well as freeing your hands to make the knots. The ends can be tied between two posts. Alternatively, you could try the "backstrap" method. Attach the start of the threads to a fixed point and the other end onto a belt around your waist.

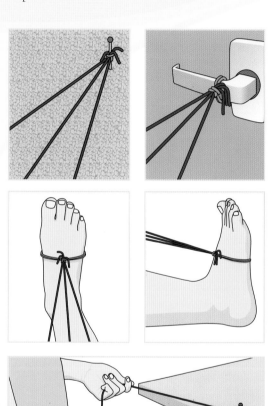

BUTTERFLY

Working with long lengths of thread can be troublesome, and you may find them easier to use if you wind them into a "butterfly." This technique can also be used to help keep several strands in the same group together.

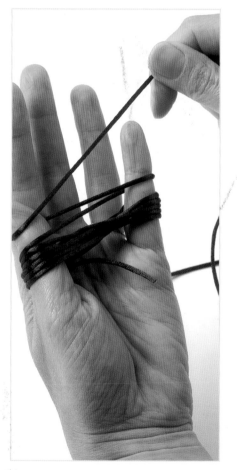

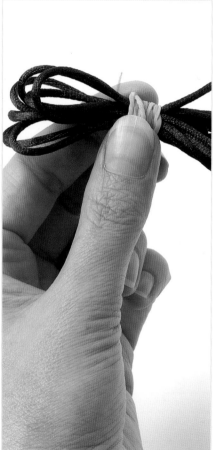

Wind the threads in a figure-eight around your thumb and little finger.

Secure them with an elastic band at the center.

OVERHAND KNOT

This is one of the most basic of knots, and it is sometimes known as a simple knot. It can be made with a single element, or worked over a core element.

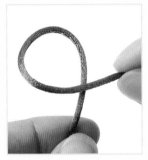 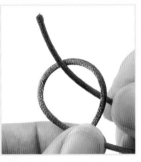 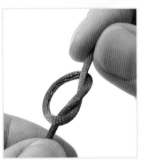

1 Make a loop so that the start of the element is lower than the end.

2 Take the end of the element behind the loop and bring it up through the loop.

3 Tighten the knot by pulling on the end.

CONNECTING OVERHAND KNOTS

A series of overhand knots can be connected together to form a length of narrow ware.

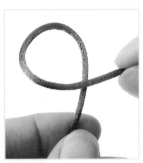 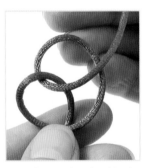

1 Make a loop so that the start of the element is lower than the end.

2 Make a new loop by taking the end of the element behind the first loop and up through it.

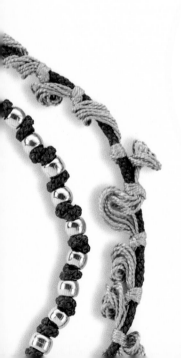

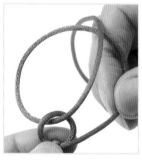

3 Tighten the first loop by pulling on the upper part of that loop.

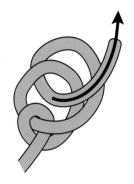

4 Make another new loop by taking the end of the element behind and up through the previous loop. Tighten the previous loop by pulling the upper part of that loop. Continue by repeating Step 4.

OVERHAND KNOTS OVER A CORE

Connected overhand knots can be worked around a second element, which forms a core.

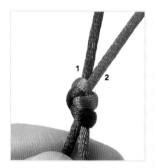

1 Tie your threads together and arrange them so that Element 1 is on the left and Element 2 is on the right. Element 1 forms the core.

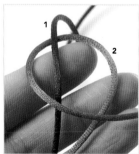

2 Make a loop around the core by taking Element 2 behind Element 1 and in front of Element 2.

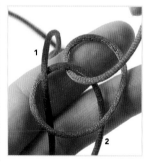

3 Finish the overhand knot by taking Element 2 through the loop from behind. Repeat Steps 2 and 3 until the required length has been made.

HALF HITCHES

Interesting narrow wares can be made by working a series of half hitches in different combinations. Half hitches are made with two elements. There are four different methods, and they can go either clockwise or counterclockwise around one of the elements.

RIGHT-HAND OVER

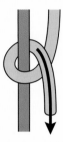

Keep the left-hand element taut and work with the element on the right. Take it over the left-hand one, up behind the left, and down over itself.

RIGHT-HAND UNDER

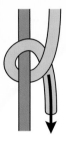

Keep the left-hand element taut and work with the element on the right. Take it under the left-hand one, up in front of the left, and down behind itself.

LEFT-HAND OVER

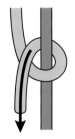

Keep the right-hand element taut and work with the element on the left. Take it over the right-hand one, up behind the right, and down over itself.

LEFT-HAND UNDER

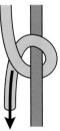

Keep the right-hand element taut and work with the element on the left. Take it under the right-hand one, up in front of the right, and down behind itself.

TIP

These samples are best worked with the start of the threads attached to a fixed point so that you can pull the elements taut. Either attach the elements directly, or use a piece of spare thread to join the elements to the fixed point. Some elements need to be kept taut at all times. If this is the case, you could tie both ends of these elements, using one of the methods described on page 30.

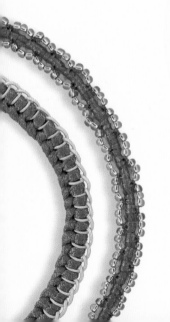

A SERIES OF IDENTICAL HALF HITCHES

Tie your elements together and arrange them so that Element 1 starts on the left. Keep this element taut at all times. Element 2 starts on the right. It has various names such as corkscrew bar, Chinese staircase, and Helter Skelter. The version with loose tension is known as a buttonhole bar.

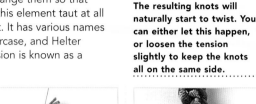

TIP
The resulting knots will naturally start to twist. You can either let this happen, or loosen the tension slightly to keep the knots all on the same side.

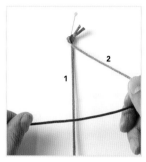

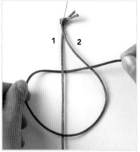

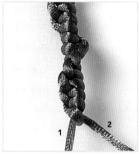

1 Start making a series of Right-hand Over hitches by taking Element 2 over Element 1, forming a loop on the right-hand side.

2 Now take it behind Element 1 and up into the loop from behind.

3 Tighten the knot and repeat from Step 2.

A SERIES OF OPPOSITE HALF HITCHES

These are also known as tatted bars. Tie your elements together and arrange them so that Element 1 starts on the left. Keep this element taut at all times. Element 2 starts on the right.

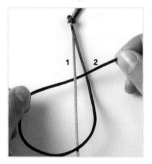

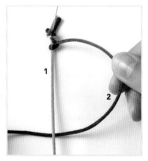

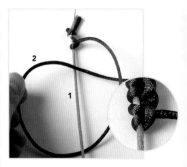

1 Start making a Right-hand Over hitch by taking Element 2 over Element 1, forming a loop on the right-hand side. Take Element 2 behind Element 1 and up into the loop from behind.

2 Tighten the knot. Start making a Right-hand Under hitch by taking Element 2 behind Element 1, forming a loop on the right-hand side.

3 Take Element 2 in front of Element 1 and down into the loop. Tighten the knot. Repeat Steps 1 to 3 until the required length has been made.

A SERIES OF LEFT- AND RIGHT-HAND HALF HITCHES

Here the two elements take it in turns to make the hitches. Only secure the start of the elements, as they both alternate between passive and working. This creates a zig-zag effect, known as single chain, single chain of seesaw knots, or single tatted chain.

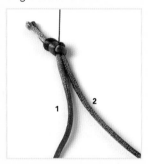

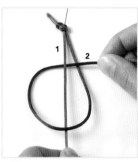

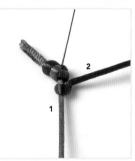

1 Tie your elements together and arrange them so that Element 1 starts on the left, and Element 2 is on the right.

2 Start making a Right-hand Over hitch (see page 34) by taking Element 2 over Element 1, forming a loop on the right-hand side. Take Element 2 behind Element 1 and up into the loop from behind.

3 Gently tighten the knot.

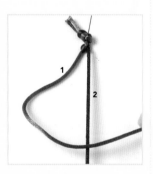

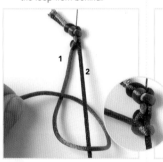

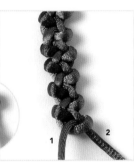

4 Keeping Element 2 taut, start making a Left-hand Over hitch (see page 34) by taking Element 1 over Element 2, forming a loop on the left-hand side.

5 Take Element 1 behind Element 2 and up into the loop from behind. Gently tighten the knot.

6 Repeat Steps 2 to 5 until the required length has been made.

A SERIES OF LEFT- AND RIGHT-HAND HALF HITCHES OVER A CORE

Working the hitches over a core element gives the narrow ware more stability.
The result is known as a single Genoese Bar.

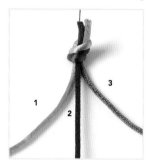

1. Tie your elements together and arrange them so that Element 1 starts on the left, Element 2 is in the middle, and Element 3 is on the right. Keep the central Element 2 taut at all times to form a core thread.

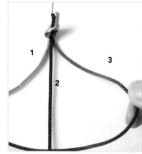

2. Start making a Right-hand Over hitch (see page 34) by taking Element 3 over Element 2, forming a loop on the right-hand side.

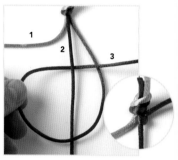

3. Now take Element 3 behind Element 2 and up into the loop from behind. Tighten the knot.

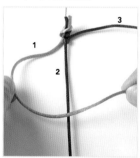

4. Start making a Left-hand Over hitch (see page 34) by taking Element 1 over Element 2, forming a loop on the left-hand side.

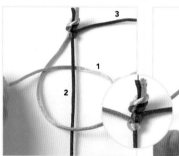

5. Now take Element 1 behind Element 2 and up into the loop from behind. Tighten the knot.

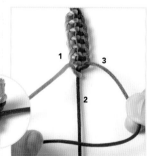

6. Repeat Steps 2 to 5 until the required length has been made.

DOUBLE LEFT- AND RIGHT-HAND HALF HITCHES OVER A CORE

Here again alternate hitches are worked over a core. As two hitches are made on each side, it creates a double Genoese Bar. The single Genoese bar is shown on page 37.

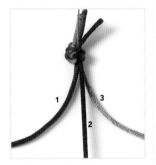

1 Tie your elements together and arrange them so that Element 1 starts on the left, Element 2 is in the middle, and Element 3 is on the right.

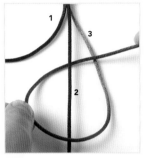

2 Start making a Right-hand Over hitch (see page 34) by taking Element 3 over Element 2, forming a loop on the right-hand side. Now take Element 3 behind Element 2 and up into the loop from behind.

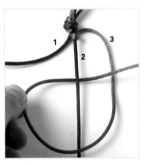

3 Tighten the knot. Repeat Step 2 so that there are two Right-hand Over hitches over Element 2.

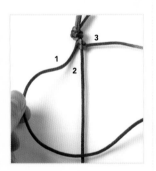

4 Start making a Left-hand Over hitch (see page 34) by taking Element 1 over Element 2, forming a loop on the left-hand side (as shown). Complete the hitch by taking Element 1 behind Element 2 and up into the loop for behind. Tighten the knot.

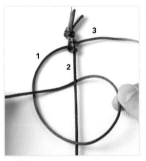

5 Repeat Step 4 so that there are two left-hand hitches over Element 2.

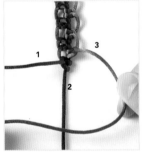

6 Repeat Steps 2 to 5 until the required length has been made.

TIP
Keep the central Element 2 taut at all times as this will form a core thread underneath the hitches.

DOUBLE LEFT- AND RIGHT-HAND OPPOSITE HALF HITCHES OVER A CORE

Yet again alternate elements are working, each making a pair of hitches over a core. However, these half hitches are not identical, but opposite. This makes a more symmetric result known as a double tatted bar.

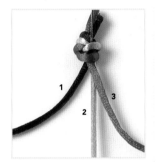

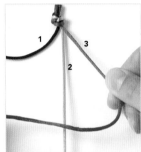

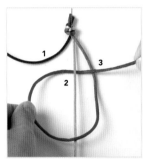

1 Tie your elements together and arrange them so that Element 1 starts on the left, Element 2 is in the middle, and Element 3 is on the right. Keep the central Element 2 taut.

2 Start making a Right-hand Over hitch (see page 34) by taking Element 3 over Element 2, forming a loop on the right-hand side.

3 Now take Element 3 behind Element 2, up into the loop from behind, and tighten the knot.

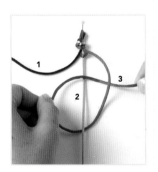

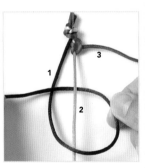

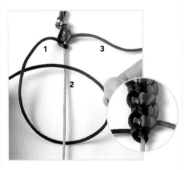

4 Start making a Right-hand Under hitch (see page 34) by taking Element 3 behind Element 2, forming a loop on the right-hand side. Then take Element 3 in front of Element 2, down into the loop, and tighten the knot.

5 Start making a Left-hand Over hitch (see page 34) by taking Element 1 over Element 2, forming a loop on the left-hand side. Now take Element 1 behind Element 2, up into the loop from behind, and tighten the knot.

6 Start making a Left-hand Under hitch (see page 34) by taking Element 1 behind Element 2, forming a loop on the left-hand side. Take Element 1 in front of Element 2, down into the loop, and tighten the knot. Repeat Steps 2 to 6 until the required length has been made.

HALF KNOTS

Half knots come into the category of macramé or square knotting. They are made from two elements that work equally, and can be made more solid by working over a third core element. A series of half knots can be worked to form a length of narrow ware.

LEFT-HAND OVER

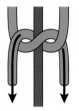

LEFT-HAND UNDER

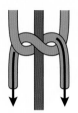

There are two forms of half knot. One is made with the left-hand element going over the right-hand element, while the other is made the opposite way around. You will find that after making a half knot, the positions of the working elements have changed over, so that if Element 1 starts on the left-hand side, it will end up on the right-hand side.

A SERIES OF IDENTICAL HALF KNOTS OVER A CORE

A series of identical half knots will create a spiral structure. It is easiest to work with all the elements secured at one end. If you wish, you can also secure the other end of the core element.

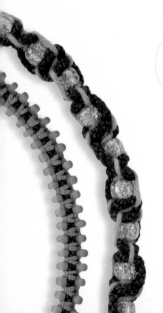

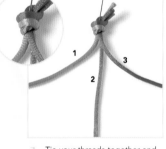

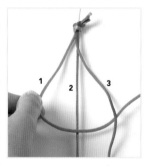

1. Tie your threads together and arrange them so that Element 1 is on the left, Element 2 is in the middle, and Element 3 is on the right. Keep the central Element 2 taut at all times. This will form the core thread underneath the half knots.

2. Make a loop on the left-hand side by taking the leftmost element over the top of the central core and under the thread on the right. (The first time you do this you will be taking Element 1 over Element 2 and under Element 3.)

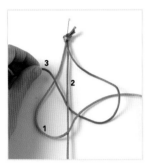 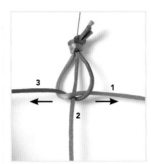 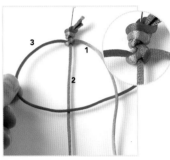

3 Now take the element that was on the right behind the core and up through the loop on the left-hand side. (The first time you do this you will be taking Element 3 behind Element 2 and up through the loop of Element 1.)

4 Tighten the knot by pulling on both the working elements in the directions shown.

5 Notice that the elements have changed places, so that Element 1 is now on the right, and Element 3 is on the left. The core thread in the middle (Element 2) is passive and has not moved. Make the next half knot in exactly the same way, by repeating Steps 2 to 4, but start with Element 3 on the left-hand side.

6 Repeat Steps 2 to 5 until the required length has been made. Always start with the leftmost element, regardless of its color.

TIP
You will find the work starts to twist. Don't try to force it straight, but let it spiral round. Don't worry if this switches the position of the elements—everything will be okay if you always make the loop with the left-hand element.

A SERIES OF OPPOSITE HALF KNOTS OVER A CORE

Here is another version of half knots worked over a core. This is a series of opposite
half knots that produces a flat structure instead of a spiral.

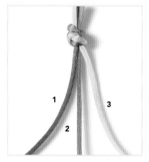

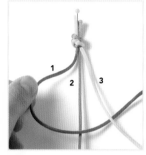

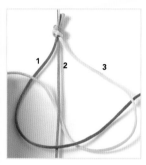

1. Tie your threads together and arrange them so that Element 1 is on the left, Element 2 is in the middle, and Element 3 is on the right. Keep the central Element 2 taut at all times as this will form the core thread underneath the half knots.

2. Make a loop on the left-hand side by taking the leftmost element (Element 1) over the top of the central core element (Element 2) and under the element on the right (Element 3).

3. Now take the element that was on the right (Element 3) behind the core and up through the loop on the left-hand side.

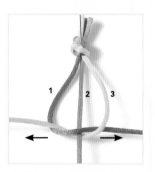

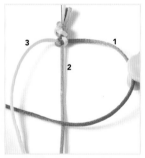

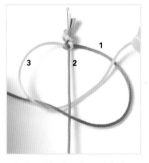

4. Tighten the knot by pulling on both the working elements in the directions shown. Notice that the elements have changed places, so that Element 1 is now on the right, and Element 3 is on the left.

5. Start making an opposite half knot. Make a loop on the right-hand side by taking the rightmost element (Element 1) over the top of the central core (Element 2) and under the element on the left (Element 3).

6. Now take the element that was on the left (Element 3) behind the core and up through the loop on the right-hand side.

TIP

The loop is always made with the same element as it shifts from side to side. If your working elements are different colors, then it is easy to keep track of which side to start the loop. However, if both of the working elements are the same color, this can be confusing. If you are not sure which side to start from, look for the element that is coming up from underneath a bump and make your loop from that one.

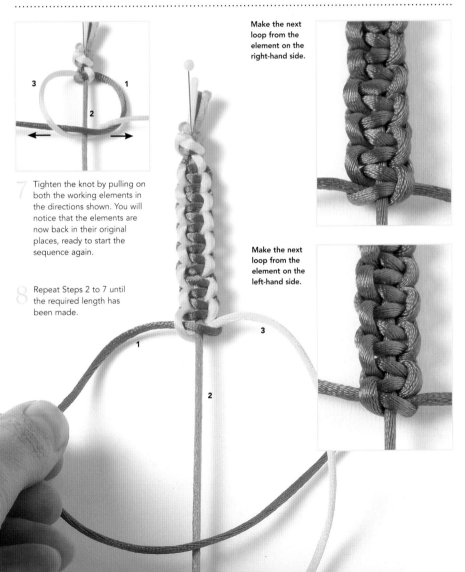

Make the next loop from the element on the right-hand side.

7 Tighten the knot by pulling on both the working elements in the directions shown. You will notice that the elements are now back in their original places, ready to start the sequence again.

8 Repeat Steps 2 to 7 until the required length has been made.

Make the next loop from the element on the left-hand side.

CROWN SINNETS

Crown sinnets are usually made with four elements. Each element works equally, going over and under adjacent elements. The knotting is supported in the hand. It may take a while to feel comfortable with the movements, especially when the four elements need to be tightened evenly.

A SERIES OF IDENTICAL CROWNS

Working identical crowns creates a firm knotted sinnet that has a round cross-section.

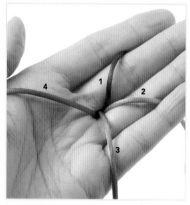

1. Tie the elements together and arrange them so that Element 1 is in the North, Element 2 is in the East, Element 3 is in the South, and Element 4 is in the West.

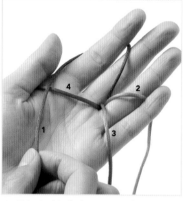

2. Take the North element over the West element. Keep a loop of the North element protruding out to the right.

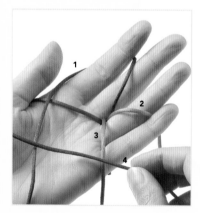

3. Take the West element over both the element just moved and the South element, so that it jumps over two elements in a counterclockwise direction.

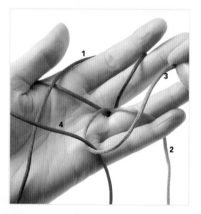

4. Take the South element over both the element just moved and the East element, so that it jumps over two elements in a counterclockwise direction.

TIP
You can try holding the growing sinnet down in your left hand between your ring and middle fingers. Then either make moves flat in hand or take the element around your fingers. You might find it faster to pinch the work in your fingertips, but that can be more difficult. Experiment with different ways of holding the work, as you may find a way that suits you better..

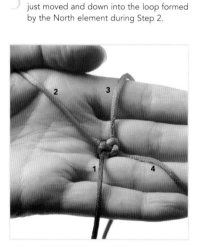

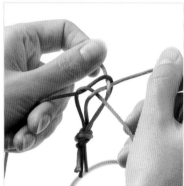

5 Take the East element over the element just moved and down into the loop formed by the North element during Step 2.

6 Tighten all the elements simultaneously by pulling them with your fingers.

8 Repeat Steps 2 to 7 until the required length has been made. Try to tighten the work evenly by pulling all four elements simultaneously in the directions shown by the arrows.

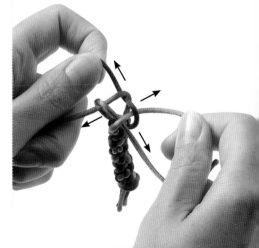

7 The elements have all shifted position by a quarter turn in a counterclockwise direction. However, from now on it does not matter where the elements start, so place any element in the North position.

A SERIES OF OPPOSITE CROWNS

Here the crowning is made alternately in a clockwise, then a counterclockwise direction. This creates a four-sided result.

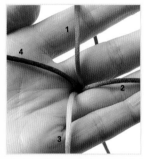

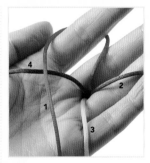

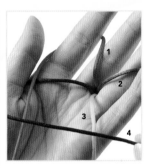

1 Tie the elements together and arrange them so that Element 1 is in the North, Element 2 is in the East, Element 3 is in the South, and Element 4 is in the West.

2 Take the North element over the West element. Keep a loop of the North element protruding out to the right.

3 Take the West element over both the element just moved and the South element, so that it jumps over two elements in a counterclockwise direction.

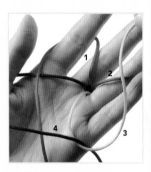

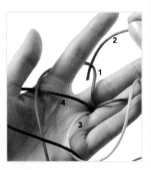

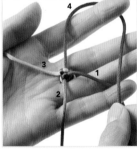

4 Take the South element over both the element just moved and the East element, so that it jumps over two elements in a counterclockwise direction.

5 Take the East element over the element just moved and down into the loop formed by the North element during Step 2. Tighten all the elements simultaneously by pulling them with your fingers.

6 Place any element in the North position. Work in the opposite (clockwise) direction. Take the North element over the East element. Keep a loop of the North element protruding out to the left.

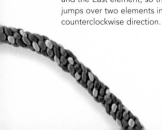

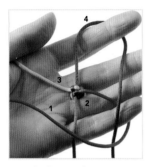

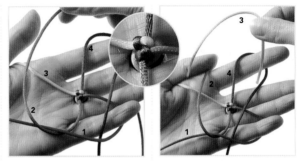

7 Take the East element over both the element just moved and the South element, so that it jumps over two elements in a clockwise direction.

8 Take the South element over both the element just moved and the West element, so that it jumps over two elements in a clockwise direction.

9 Take the West element over the element just moved and down into the loop formed by the North element during Step 6. Tighten all the elements simultaneously by pulling them with your fingers.

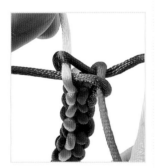

10 Continue working making a counterclockwise crown (Steps 2 to 5), followed by a clockwise crown (Steps 6 to 9). Repeat until the required length has been made.

TIP
If you are not sure which way you should be going, check these photographs.

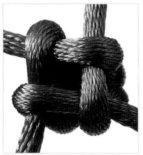

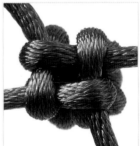

Ready to crown in a clockwise direction (from Step 6)

Ready to crown in a counterclockwise direction (from Step 2)

Interlooping

Interlooping can be made with one or more elements and covers techniques such as crochet and knitting. Simple narrow wares using one or two loops can easily be made with your fingers. There are many ways of holding the elements as you make the moves and the illustrations here show you one way for each method. However, when you feel confident with the process, you can try experimenting with several different methods to see which suits you better.

EQUIPMENT

Instead of your fingers, you can use equipment, such as the two-pronged tool known as a "lucet," "lyre," or "chain fork." There are many wooden or bone antique examples to be found, as well as modern plastic versions.

A lucet usually has a small hole in its central body. Most instructions will tell you to put the thread through the hole. However, this is a fallacy and causes a lot of problems as the hole is usually too small to accommodate the work.

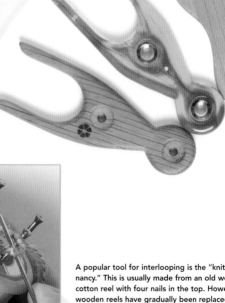

A popular tool for interlooping is the "knitting nancy." This is usually made from an old wooden cotton reel with four nails in the top. However, as wooden reels have gradually been replaced with plastic ones, they now have to be specially made. A needle is used to ease the loops over the prongs. Sometimes, you will find tools with more than four prongs. These "knitting spools," or "moule turcs" work in the same way as the knitting nancy, except they use more loops, creating a wider piece of tubular knitting.

ONE ELEMENT, ONE LOOP

This is the minimum requirement for interlooping and can be swiftly made using your fingers. However, you could also use a crochet hook as it is the basic single chain of crochet.

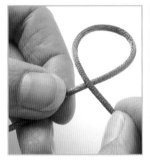

1 Make a loop so that the start of the element is lower than the end.

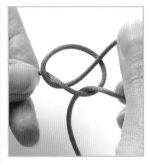

2 Pull another loop up through this loop and tighten it by pulling the new loop.

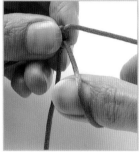

3 Hold the start of the work in your left hand. With your right-hand thumb and index finger, open up the loop and grab the end of the element.

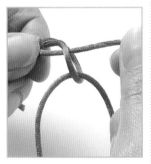

4 Make a new loop by pulling up the element from below. Pull the new loop to tighten the old one.

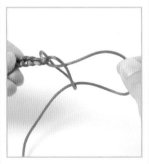

5 Repeat Steps 3 and 4 until the required length is made.

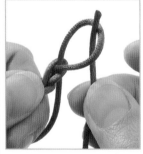

6 To finish, take the end of the element right through the last loop and tighten it to close the loop.

ONE ELEMENT, TWO LOOPS (FOR LUCET)

Two loops can easily be controlled over your fingers, although they are
more often worked on a tool called a "lucet." You can build up quite a bit
of speed when using a tool that has been especially designed for a job.

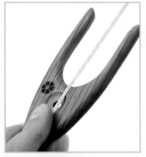

1 With your left hand, hold the
start of the element against the
back of the lucet. You will need
to hold it down for several
movements until it
is stable.

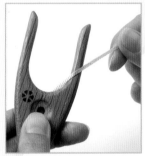

2 Now wrap the rest of the
element in a figure-eight
around the prongs. Bring the
element to the front and take it
counterclockwise around the
right-hand prong.

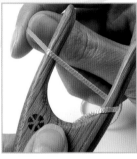

3 From the back of the right-
hand prong, take it to the front
of the left-hand prong.

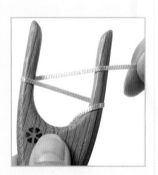

4 Go clockwise around the
left-hand prong and bring it
from behind the left-hand
prong to the front of the
right-hand prong.

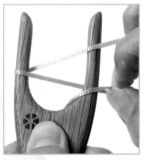

5 With your middle to little
fingers, hold the working end
of the element to the back of
the right-hand prong, so that it
rests on the top part of the
prong. With your thumb and
index finger, pick up the lower
loop that is sitting around the
lower part of the prong.

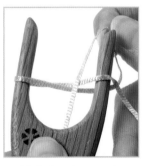

6 Lift this lower loop over the
working end and off the prong.
The working end has now
formed a new loop around
the prong.

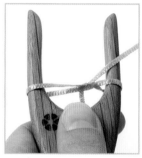

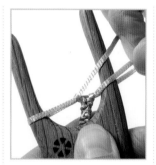

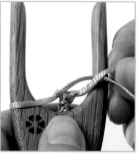

7 Turn the lucet in the palm of your left hand, so that the right-hand prong goes over the left-hand one. Tighten the stitch by pulling the working end toward the right.

8 Repeat from Step 5 until the required length has been made.

9 To finish, take the working end right through the loop on the right-hand prong. Lift the loop off the prong and tighten to close the loop.

10 Repeat the process for the loop on the left-hand side.

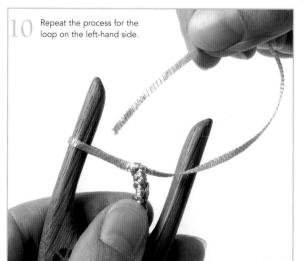

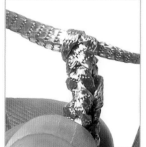

Close up after Step 9

TIP
If you find it difficult to lift the loops off the prongs, use a blunt needle to ease them off.

ONE ELEMENT, TWO LOOPS (FOR FINGERS)

You can create two loops with your fingers—the advantage of fingers is that they are always to hand!

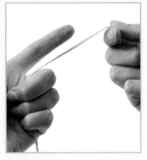

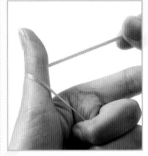

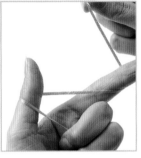

1 Hold the start of the element in the palm of your left hand with your middle to little fingers. You will need to hold it down for several movements until it is stable.

2 Bring the element to the front of your thumb, then clockwise around to the back of the thumb.

3 Bring the element to the front of your index finger, then counterclockwise around to the back.

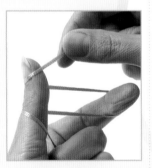

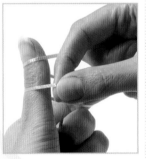

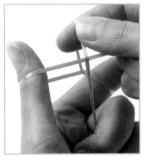

4 Bring the element to the back of your thumb, then counterclockwise around to the front of the thumb, so that it rests above the loop already around the thumb.

5 With your middle to little fingers on your right hand, hold the working end of the element. With your right thumb and index finger, pick up the lower loop that is sitting around the thumb.

6 Lift this lower loop over the working end and off the thumb. The working end has now formed a new loop around the finger. Tighten the stitch by pulling the working end to the right.

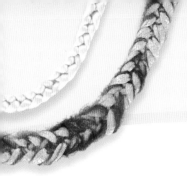

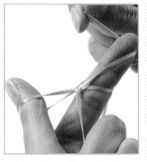

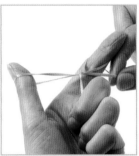

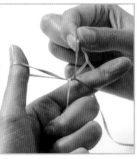

7 Take the working end in front of the left index finger and counterclockwise around to the back, so that it rests above the loop already on the finger.

8 Hold the working end in the lower fingers of the right hand and pick up the lower loop with the index finger and thumb of the right hand.

9 Lift the lower loop over the working end and off the finger. Tighten the stitch by pulling the working end toward the left.

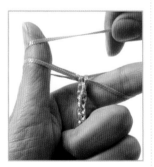

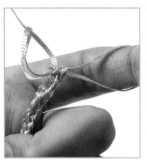

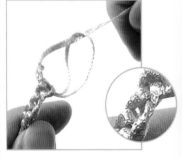

10 Repeat from Steps 4 to 9, tensioning the finished work downward in the palm of the left hand.

11 To finish, take the end of the element right through the loop on your thumb.

12 Lift the loop off your thumb and pull the end of the element to close the loop. Repeat this process for the loop on your index finger.

ONE ELEMENT, TWO LOOPS WITH HITCHES

Making hitches with the element changes the structure. The instructions are the same for working on your fingers or a lucet (just replace the word finger with prong).

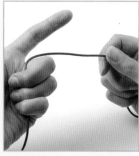

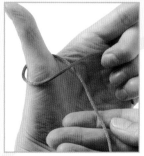

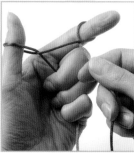

1 Hold the start of the element in the palm of your left hand with your middle to little fingers. You will need to hold it down for several movements until it is stable.

2 Twist a loop to the left so that the working end is lower and forward of the other end. Place this loop over your left thumb.

3 Twist a loop to the right, so that the working end is lower and forward of the other end. Put this loop on your left index finger.

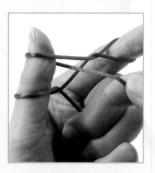

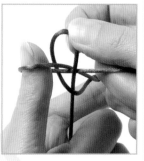

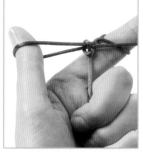

4 Twist a loop to the left so that the working end is lower and forward of the other end. Put this on your left thumb so that it sits above the loop that is already there.

5 Lift the lower loop over the one above and off the thumb.

6 Tighten the stitch by pulling the working end to the right, in front of the index finger.

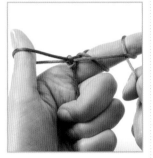

7 Twist a loop to the right so that the working end is lower and forward of the other end. Put this loop on your left index finger, above the one already there.

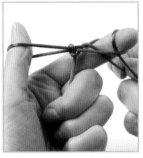

8 Lift the lower loop over the one above and off the finger.

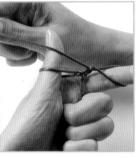

9 Tighten the stitch by pulling the working end to the left.

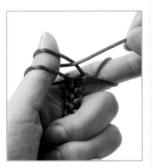

10 Repeat from Steps 4 to 9, tensioning the work downward in the palm of your hand.

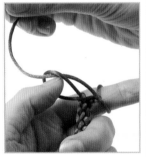

11 To finish, take the end of the element right through the loop on the thumb. Lift the loop off the thumb and pull the end to close the loop.

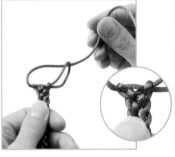

12 Take the end right through the loop on the index finger. Take the loop off the finger and pull the end to tighten the stitch.

ONE ELEMENT, FOUR LOOPS: ROUND

It is possible to work four loops on your fingers. The tensioning tends to make large stitches so it is more suited to chunkier yarns. Finer samples can be made using equipment. The instructions show a specially made wooden spool being used, giving rise to the term "spool knitting." A tapestry needle is also used to help with the lifting of the loops. These are the instructions for making the classic "French knitting," a tubular knitted structure.

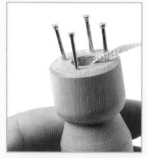

1 Thread the start of the element through the spool.

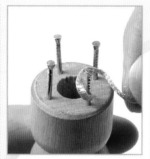

2 Hold the start of the element at the base of the spool with your left hand. Take the working end of the element in your right hand and take it clockwise around the peg closest to you.

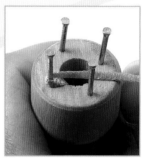

3 Turn the spool a quarter turn clockwise and take the working end inside of the next peg.

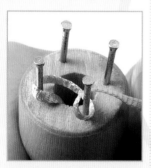

4 Turn the element clockwise around this peg.

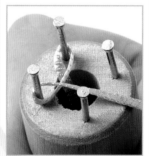

5 Turn the spool a quarter turn clockwise and take the working end inside of the next peg.

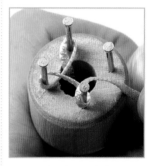

6 Turn the element clockwise around this peg.

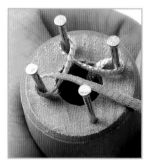

7 Turn the spool a quarter turn clockwise and take the working end inside of the next peg.

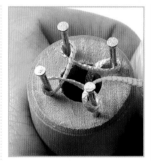

8 Turn the element clockwise around this peg. All of the pegs should now have a loop around them.

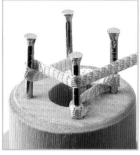

9 Turn the spool a quarter turn clockwise and take the working element in front of the next peg so that it sits above the loop already on the peg.

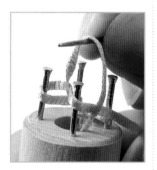

10 Using the tapestry needle, lift the lower loop over the element and off the peg. The working element is now making the new loop.

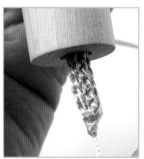

11 Repeat Steps 9 and 10. Tension the work by pulling on the start of the element at the base of the spool.

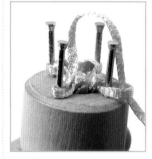

12 To finish, take the working end right through each loop before lifting them off the pegs. Tighten the stitches by pulling the end.

ONE ELEMENT, FOUR LOOPS: FLAT

A similar principle can be used to make a flat version of "spool knitting." This can also be worked over your fingers, but the result will have a looser tension.

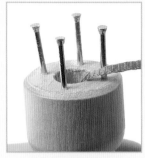

1. Thread the start of the element through the spool and hold it at the base with your left hand.

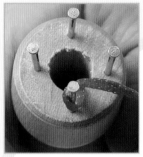

2. Hold the working end of the element in your right hand and take it clockwise around the first peg.

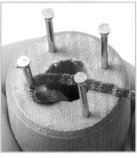

3. Turn the spool a quarter turn clockwise and take the working end inside of the next peg.

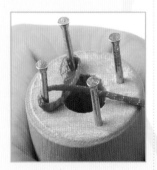

4. Turn the element clockwise around this second peg. Turn the spool a quarter turn clockwise and take the working end inside of the next peg.

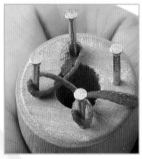

5. Turn the element clockwise around this third peg.

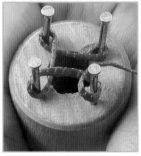

6. Turn the spool a quarter turn clockwise and take the working end inside of the next peg. Turn the element clockwise around this fourth peg. All of the pegs should have a loop around them.

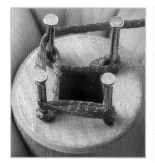

7 Take the element clockwise, back around the outside of the four pegs. There should be nothing between the first and fourth peg.

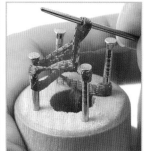

8 Lift the lower loops over the element and off the pegs, starting with the fourth and working back round to the first peg.

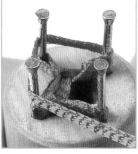

9 Take the element counterclockwise, back around the outside of the four pegs.

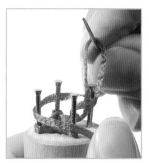

10 Lift the lower loops over the element and off the pegs, starting with the first and working back around to the fourth peg.

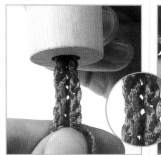

11 Continue working by repeating Steps 7 to 10. Tension the work by pulling on the start of the element at the base of the spool.

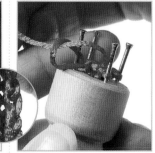

12 To finish, take the working end right through each loop before lifting them off the pegs. Tighten the stitches by pulling the end.

TWO ELEMENTS, ONE LOOP

Here two elements are worked together by taking them alternately
through a single loop. These techniques are easily made in the hand
because only one loop needs to be maintained. You can see why this first
version is often called "finger knitting," as the index fingers act like two
knitting needles.

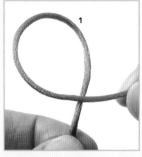

1 Make a loop in Element 1 so
that the start of the element is
lower than the end.

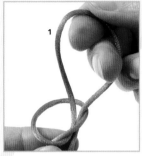

2 Still working with Element 1,
pull another loop up through
this loop and tighten it by
pulling the new loop.

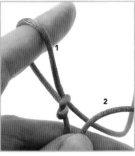

3 Put this loop on your left index
finger and hold the start of
both Element 1 and 2 between
your left thumb and middle
finger, with Element 2 sitting
out to the right.

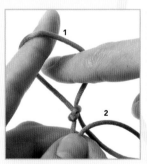

4 Take your right-hand index
finger into the loop, going from
the hand toward the fingertip.

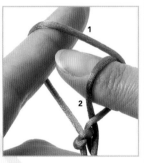

5 Using the back of the right
index finger, pick up a loop of
Element 2.

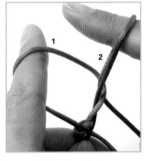

6 With the right index finger,
draw Element 2 up through the
loop so that it forms a new
loop on the right index finger.

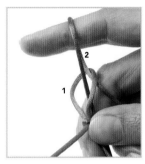

7 Exchange the start of the work from the left to right hand. Release the loop on the left finger and tighten it by pulling on the end of Element 1.

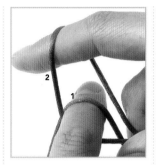

8 Take your left-hand index finger into the loop on the right hand, going from the hand toward the fingertip and pick up Element 1 on the back of your left finger.

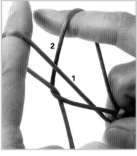

9 With the left index finger, draw Element 1 up through the loop so that it forms a new loop on the left index finger.

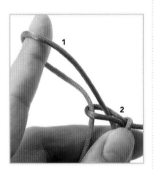

10 Exchange the start of the work from the right to left hand. Release the loop on the right finger and tighten it by pulling on the end of Element 2.

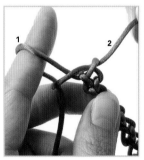

11 Repeat Steps 4 to 10 until the required length has been made.

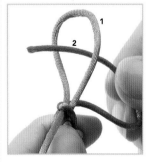

12 To finish, take the end of Element 2 right through the last loop and tighten to close the loop.

TWO ELEMENTS, ONE LOOP: TRIANGULAR

This is another version using two elements and one loop. The result is more triangular than that of the previous round one.

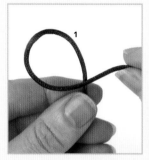

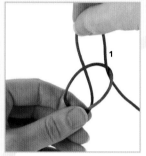

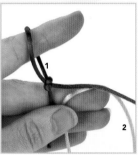

1 Make a loop in Element 1 so that the start of the element is lower than the end.

2 Still working with Element 1, pull another loop up through this loop. Tighten it by pulling the new loop.

3 Place the loop on your left index finger and hold the start of both Element 1 and Element 2 between your left thumb and middle finger.

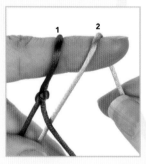

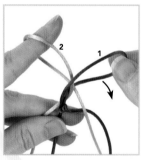

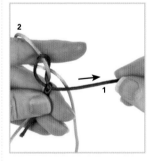

4 Take Element 2 in your right hand, making sure it goes under Element 1. Take it over the top of your left index finger so that it sits closer to the tip than the loop in Element 1.

5 Lift the loop in Element 1 over Element 2 and off the finger.

6 Tighten the stitch by pulling the end of Element 1 with your right hand.

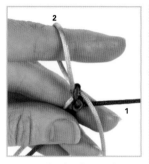

7 Note that the elements have now swapped places.

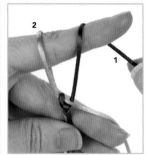

8 Now take Element 1 in your right hand, making sure it goes behind Element 2. Take Element 1 over the tip of your left index finger.

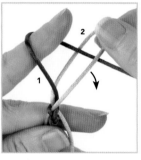

9 Lift the loop in Element 2 over Element 1 and off the finger.

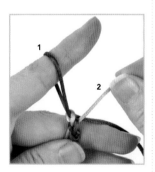

10 Tighten the stitch by pulling the end of Element 2.

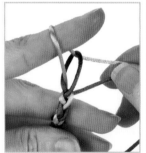

11 Continue working Steps 4 to 10 tensioning the growing work between your left thumb and middle finger.

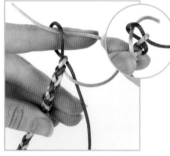

12 To finish, take the element right through the last loop before lifting it off the finger. Pull the end of the other element to close the loop.

TWO ELEMENTS, TWO LOOPS

This technique can be worked on your fingers or a lucet—the instructions are the same for both. Two loops are used, with each element being worked through its own loop. In fact, they are two chain sinnets (one element, one loop) connecting together with a cross at the center.

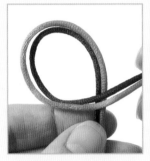

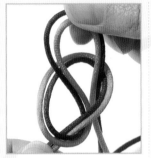

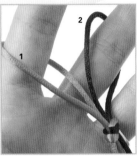

1 Hold both elements together and work them as a single element, making a loop so that the start of the element is lower than the end.

2 Still working with both elements as one, pull another loop up through the previous loop and tighten it by pulling the new loop.

3 Now divide the elements and put Element 1 on your left index finger and Element 2 on your left middle finger.

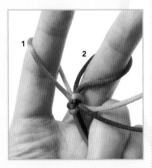

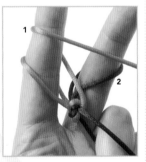

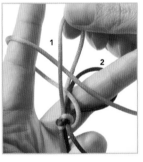

4 Hold the start of the elements underneath your ring and little finger. Make sure that the working end of Element 1 is on the right-hand side and underneath the working end of Element 2. You may find it more comfortable to hold the work between the thumb and the fourth or little finger as shown in Step 10.

5 Make a new loop on the left index finger by bringing Element 1 up between the fingers and counterclockwise around the back of the index finger, so that it rests at the tip of the finger.

6 Lift the previous, (lower) loop over the element and off the finger.

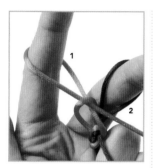

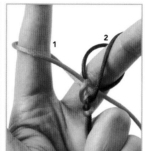

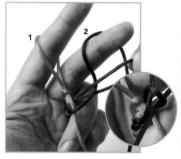

7 Pull the end of Element 1 to tighten the stitch, and make sure that it remains to the right and above Element 2.

8 Now make a new loop on the left middle finger, by taking Element 2 up between the fingers and clockwise around the back of the middle finger, so that it rests on the tip of the finger.

9 Lift the previous, lower loop over the new one and off the finger. Pull the end of Element 2 to tighten the stitch, and make sure that it remains to the left and above Element 1.

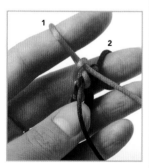

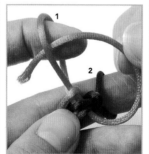

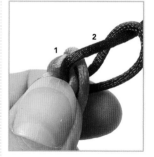

10 Continue by repeating Steps 5 to 9.

11 To finish, take the working end of Element 1 right through the loop before lifting it off your finger. Pull the end of Element 1 so that the loop closes.

12 Do the same for Element 2.

Weaving

Weaving is made from a warp and weft. The warp is a group of elements that work from the top to bottom of the weaving, running parallel to the outer edges, while the weft lies perpendicular to these edges, and works its way back and forth across the warp threads. Two is the minimum number of warps required for weaving.

EQUIPMENT

When working with two warps, it is quite convenient to make examples in the hand, without any equipment. As with twisting, knotting, and braiding, it does help to have one end of the elements attached to a fixed point, so that the sample can be held under tension.

When working with more than two warps, it is easier to have both ends of the warp elements secured. You can use two warping posts, or a "backstrap" set up like that shown on page 30.

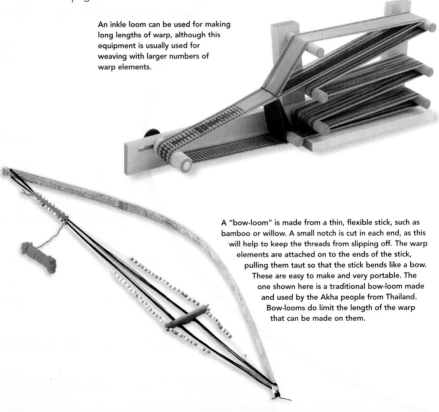

An inkle loom can be used for making long lengths of warp, although this equipment is usually used for weaving with larger numbers of warp elements.

A "bow-loom" is made from a thin, flexible stick, such as bamboo or willow. A small notch is cut in each end, as this will help to keep the threads from slipping off. The warp elements are attached on to the ends of the stick, pulling them taut so that the stick bends like a bow. These are easy to make and very portable. The one shown here is a traditional bow-loom made and used by the Akha people from Thailand. Bow-looms do limit the length of the warp that can be made on them.

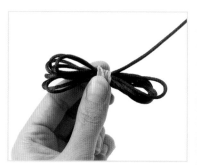

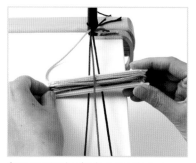

A lot of thread is required for a weft as it works its way back and forth across the weaving. Working with long lengths of thread can be troublesome, so try rolling them up and securing with an elastic band at the center. See page 31.

If you are using the "fixed warp" method, you can wind the threads onto a shuttle. These can also be helpful for lifting the warp elements as the weft passes under and over them. Shuttles are available ready-made, but you can easily cut a notch in either end of a smooth, flat piece of wood.

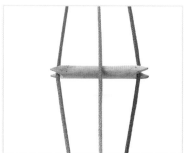

Popsicle sticks are an easy way of making a shuttle for your threads. Just cut a notch in either end.

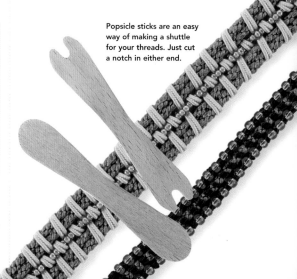

A warp spacer is a useful piece of equipment. A small stick can push apart the outer two warps, making it easier to find the space between them. A small piece of bamboo, or a plastic drinking straw will do. Cut a notch in each end, for the warp threads to sit in.

WEAVING WITH TWO WARPS: HANDHELD METHOD

Weaving with two warps and a weft can be done using a handheld method, similar to braiding. The samples are best worked with the start of the threads attached to a fixed point so that you can pull the elements taut. As the elements move around they will sit in one of three positions that you will need to identify—left, center, and right.

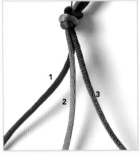

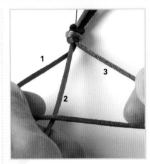

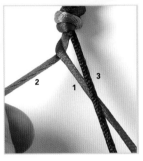

1 Tie your elements together and attach the start to a fixed point. Arrange the elements so that Element 1 (the weft) is on the left-hand side, Element 2 is in the center, and Element 3 is on the right-hand side.

2 Take the element in the left position over the element in the center.

3 Take the element in the right position over the element in the center.

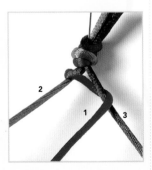

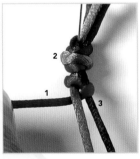

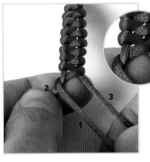

4 Take the element in the right position over the element in the center.

5 Take the element in the left position over the element in the center.

6 Repeat Steps 2 to 5 holding all the elements taut at all times. When the warp is finished, secure the ends to stop them unraveling.

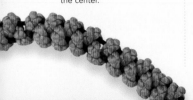

WEAVING WITH TWO WARPS: FIXED WARP METHOD

This creates the same weave structure, but is made with the warp elements secured so that they are held under tension at all times. In this case the elements are attached to warping posts with a piece of spare thread. The weft (Element 1) should only be attached at the start and should lie on the left-hand side of the warps. Make sure that Element 3 is on the right-hand side.

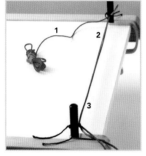

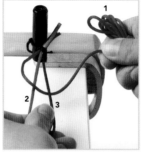

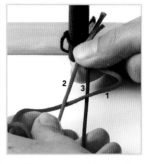

1 Tie your elements together and attach the start to a fixed point. Tie the other end of Elements 2 and 3 to another fixed point, so that they are lying taut between the two points.

2 Take the weft over Element 2 and under Element 3, so that it ends up on the right-hand side.

3 Now take the weft back to the left, going over Element 3, then under Element 2.

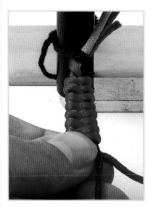

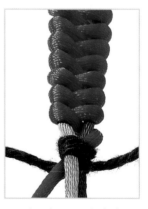

TIP
Use the left-hand thumb and index finger to pinch the work as you make a move. This helps to keep the tension even.

4 Repeat Steps 2 and 3, taking care to arrange the weft evenly over the warps.

5 When the warp is finished, secure the ends to stop them unraveling.

WEAVING WITH THREE WARPS

Weaving with more than two warps is best done with a fixed warp method. With three warps the weft turns the same way around the two outer edges of the weaving. The weft (Element 1) should only be attached at the start and should lie on the left-hand side of the warps. The warps should lie parallel so that Element 2 is on the left, Element 3 is in the center, and Element 4 is on the right.

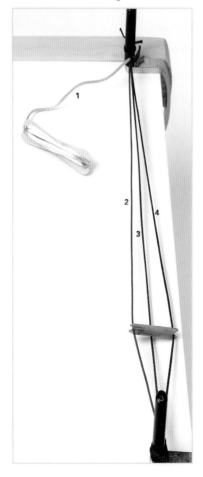

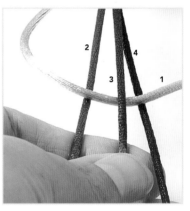

2 Take the weft over Element 2, under Element 3, and over Element 4, so that it ends up on the right-hand side.

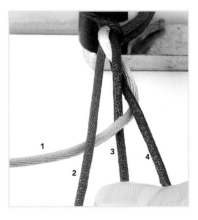

1 Tie your elements together and attach the start to a fixed point. Tie the other end of Elements 2, 3, and 4 (the warps) to another fixed point, so that the warps are lying taut between the two points.

3 Now take the weft back to the left, going under Element 4, over Element 3, and under Element 2.

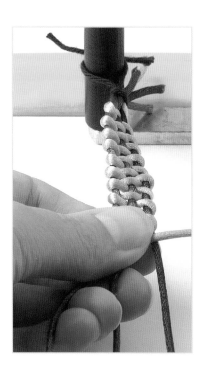

TIP

Use the left-hand thumb and index finger to pinch the work as you make a move. This helps to keep the tension even.

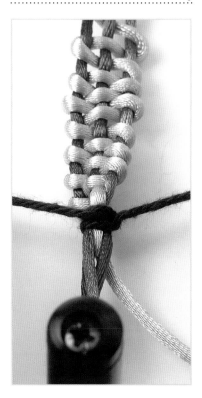

4   Repeat Steps 2 and 3, taking care to arrange the weft evenly over the warps.

TIP

This method of working can result in samples that have a tendency to twist. If you wish to straighten the work, hold the sample flat and carefully pass it over a steaming kettle or pan. Be very careful not to scald yourself.

5   When the warp is finished, secure the ends to stop them unraveling.

Braiding

A wide range of different braiding techniques have developed all over the world, including "Kumihimo" from Japan, "Slentre" from Denmark, and "Tili" from the Middle East. Braiding can be worked with any number of elements, from three or above. Although some forms can be quite complex, there are plenty of possibilities that are made with only a few elements, and these require little or no equipment.

EQUIPMENT

Working without equipment is known as "free-end braiding," "plaiting," or "sinnet making." Although it is possible to hold the work in your hand, it is easier if the start of the work is attached to a fixed point (as it is in twisting, knotting, and weaving).

Threads can be rolled onto purpose-made bobbins, such as these Kumihimo examples.

Working with long lengths of thread can be troublesome. Try rolling them up and securing with an elastic band at the center (see page 31). This technique can also be used to help keep several strands together in the same group.

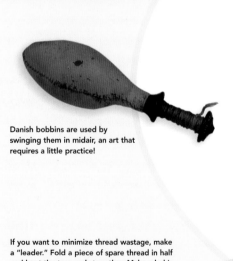

Danish bobbins are used by swinging them in midair, an art that requires a little practice!

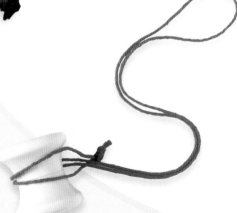

If you want to minimize thread wastage, make a "leader." Fold a piece of spare thread in half and knot the two ends together. Make a lark's head knot (shown below) with this and attach it around the bobbin. Tie the braid threads to the leader rather than directly onto the bobbin.

Bobbins can be improvised, for example by using old cotton reels. Weighted bobbins can help by providing a gentle tension on the threads, and empty film canisters can be filled with something heavy to provide some weight for tensioning the threads. A rubber band on the end of the canister forms a ridge that helps prevent the thread from slipping off the bobbin.

Lace bobbins can be used for making braids.

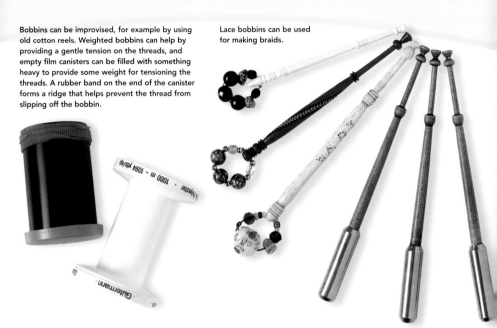

SUPPORTING THE BOBBINS

An ordinary board, pillow, or cushion can be used to support the weighted bobbins. You will need to organize your setup so that the bobbins are still providing a tension by "hanging" away from the fixed point.

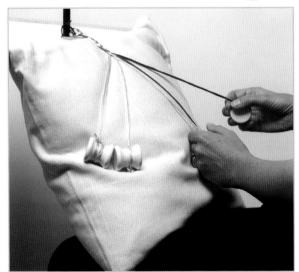

THREE-ELEMENT BRAID

This is the most common braid structure and it may surprise you that it can be made in many different ways. However, this is the most usual way, made in the same manner as plaiting hair. This braid and the four-element flat braid can both be described as plain oblique interlacing, as the elements cross over each other in an "over one, under one" fashion.

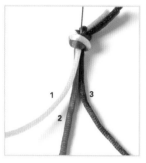

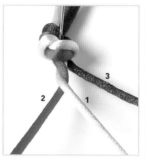

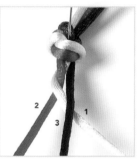

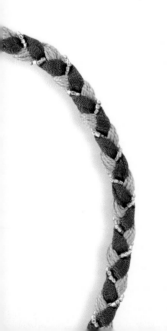

1 Join all the elements together and attach them to a fixed point. Arrange them in order so that Element 1 is on the left, Element 2 is in the center, and Element 3 is on the right.

2 Take the element on the left over the element in the center.

3 Take the element on the right over the element in the center.

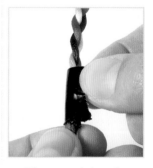

4 Do not worry that the elements are in different positions. Continue by repeating Steps 2 and 3, keeping the elements taut at all times.

5 When you reach the end, secure the elements to stop them unraveling. Here they have been temporarily secured with a piece of sticky tape.

FOUR-ELEMENT FLAT BRAID

This is a slightly wider version of the classic three-element braid. As both of the outer edges slant in the same direction, the results can have a tendency to twist. If you wish to straighten the work, hold the sample flat and carefully pass it over a steaming kettle or pan. Be careful not to scald yourself.

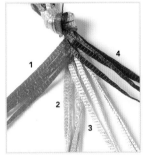

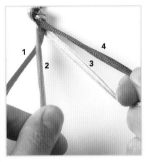

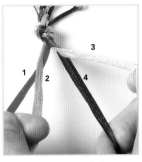

1 Tie all the elements together and attach them to a fixed point. Arrange them in order of Elements 1 to 4 from left to right.

2 Take the left-hand element over the element to its right.

3 Take the right-hand element under the element to its left.

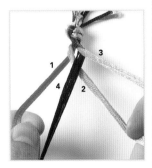

4 Cross over the two central elements, taking the right over the left.

5 Do not worry that the elements are in different positions. Continue by repeating Steps 2 to 4, keeping the elements taut at all times.

TIP
When you reach the end, secure the elements with a piece of sticky tape to stop them unraveling.

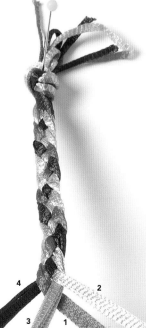

ATTACHING A STRAND TO A BOBBIN

A securing hitch is used to stop the element slipping off the bobbin.

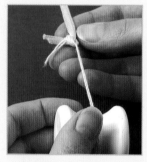

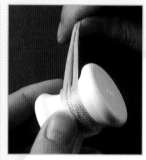

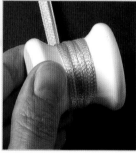

1 Knot the element onto the end of the leader. You can use a slip knot—it releases the threads easily at the end—but any knot will do. Here an overhand knot is used.

2 Wind the element onto the bobbin.

3 Now start the securing hitch by making sure that the element is coming from underneath the bobbin, up toward the fixed point.

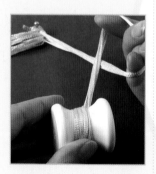

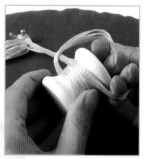

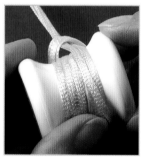

4 Make a loop in the element, making sure that the strands closest to the bobbin are uppermost.

5 Bring the bobbin up into the loop from underneath.

6 Tighten the hitch around the bobbin.

FOUR-ELEMENT ROUND BRAID

Here the four elements are worked together to produce a round braid. There are many different ways of making this structure. The method shown below can be worked with the elements held in the hand or with the elements attached to bobbins resting over a surface such as a pillow. The bobbins help to tension the braid as well as keep all the strands for one element together.

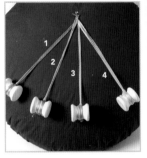

1 Tie all the elements together and attach them to a fixed point. Add bobbins to the ends of the elements and arrange them in order of Elements 1 to 4 from left to right.

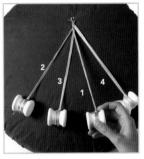

2 Take the leftmost element and move it to the right, going over two elements.

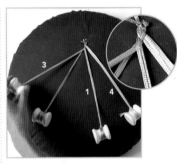

3 Take the element in the center left position and move it to the leftmost position, going over one element.

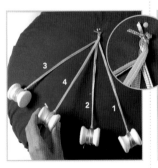

4 Take the rightmost element and move it to the left, going over two elements.

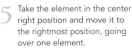

5 Take the element in the center right position and move it to the rightmost position, going over one element.

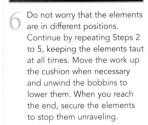

6 Do not worry that the elements are in different positions. Continue by repeating Steps 2 to 5, keeping the elements taut at all times. Move the work up the cushion when necessary and unwind the bobbins to lower them. When you reach the end, secure the elements to stop them unraveling.

TIP
Keep pairs of bobbins spread apart to improve tension.

FOUR-ELEMENT CHAIN-LINK BRAID

This is a variation of the round braid that creates a "chain-link" effect. Again there is a slight tendency for the results to twist. If you wish to straighten the work, hold the sample flat and carefully pass it over a steaming kettle or pan. Be careful not to scald yourself.

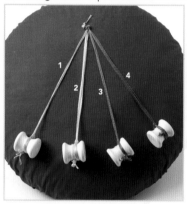

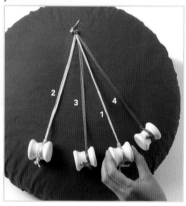

1 Tie all the elements together and attach them to a fixed point. Add bobbins onto the ends of the elements (see page 76) and arrange them in order of Elements 1 to 4 from left to right.

2 Take the leftmost element and move it to the right, going over two elements.

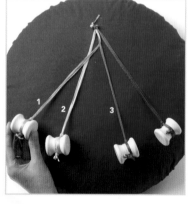

3 Take the element in the center right position (the same element moved in Step 2) and move it to the leftmost position, going under one element, then over the next.

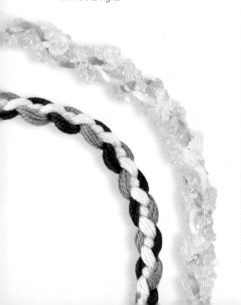

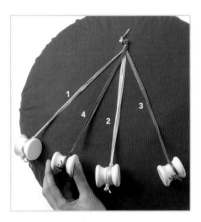

4 Take the rightmost element and take it to the left, going over two elements.

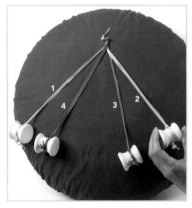

5 Take the element in the center right position and take it to the rightmost position, going over one element.

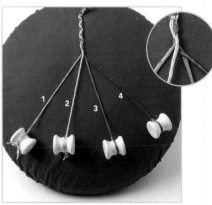

6 Continue by repeating Steps 2 to 5, keeping the elements taut at all times. Move the work up the cushion when necessary and unwind the bobbins to lower them. When you reach the end, secure the elements to stop them unraveling.

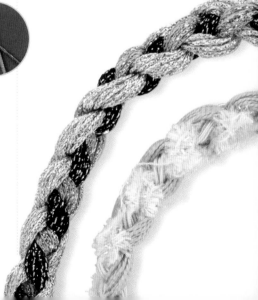

FIVE-ELEMENT, TWO-RIDGE BRAID

The two basic steps that create this braid mean that it can easily be produced using the handheld method. If you choose this option, take care to pinch the end of the braid as you work. This will help keep the tension firm and stop the braid unraveling. Alternatively, you can attach the elements to weighted bobbins and rest them over a surface.

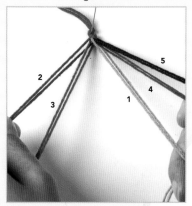

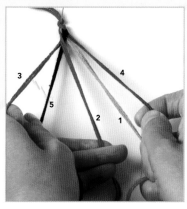

1 Tie all the elements together and attach them to a fixed point. Arrange them in order of Elements 1 to 5 from left to right, and hold Elements 1 to 3 in the left hand and the other two in the right hand. Take the leftmost element and take it to the right, going over two elements. Pinch the work in your right hand and make the move with your left hand. You should now have three elements in your right hand (as shown above).

TIP
You can keep the tension even by pinching the work in one hand, while making the move with the other.

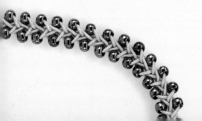

2 Take the rightmost element and take it to the left, going over two elements. You should now have three elements in your left hand. Repeat Step 1 (the photo shows Step 1 being repeated).

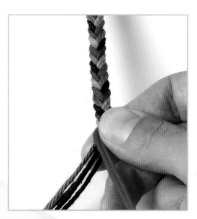

3 To make the moves pinch the work in your left hand and make the move with your right hand. Continue by repeating Steps 1 and 2, keeping the elements taut.

FIVE-ELEMENT, FOUR-RIDGE BRAID

Here the two basic steps make symmetrical "over and under" moves. It is not as easy as the two-ridge version, so you may wish to attach the elements to bobbins. If you use the hand-held method, take care to pinch the end of the braid as you work. This will help keep the tension firm and stop the braid unraveling.

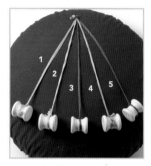

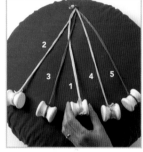

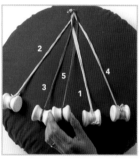

1 Tie the elements together and attach them to a fixed point. Attach the other ends onto bobbins (see page 76) and arrange them over a surface in order of Elements 1 to 5 from left to right.

2 Take the leftmost element and move it to the right, going over one element and under the next element.

3 Take the rightmost element and take it to the left, going over one element and under the next element.

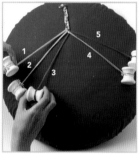

5 Continue repeating Steps 2 and 3, keeping the elements taut at all times. Move the work up the cushion when necessary and unwind the bobbins to lower them. When you reach the end, secure the elements to stop them unraveling.

4 Do not worry that the elements are in different positions. Continue repeating Steps 2 and 3, keeping the elements taut at all times. Move the work up the cushion when necessary and unwind the bobbins to lower them. When you reach the end, secure the elements to stop them unraveling.

TIP
Spread the bobbins wide apart from each other to help keep an even tension.

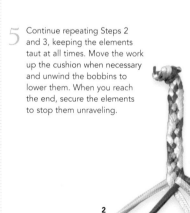

Ply-split Darning

Ply-splitting is the process of taking an element between the plies of a twisted cord. The technique can be used to make either a braid structure or a "warp twined" structure. This has similarities to weaving, in that a weft element is taken backward and forward across a set of warp elements. However, unlike weaving, where the weft goes under and over the warps, here the weft is taken through, between the plies of each warp element. Machine-made threads can be used for the warps, but a better result can be achieved by using handmade two-ply cords, such as those shown earlier in the book. The two-ply warps enable the ply-splitting to be even, with one ply sitting either side of the weft element.

EQUIPMENT

Little or no equipment is required for ply-splitting, it can be made simply by opening up the ply and pushing (or pulling) the element through by hand. Ply-splitting does not need securing while work is in progress, as the twist in the cords help to fasten each stitch as it is made. The firmer the cord, the better the stitches are secured, so be sure to put plenty of twist into your cords. Either S- or Z-twist cords can be used, or a combination of both.

A selection of tools that can be helpful for drawing the thread through the plies.
1. Tapestry needle
2. and 3. Bodkins
4. Forceps
5. Crochet hook
6. Latchet hook

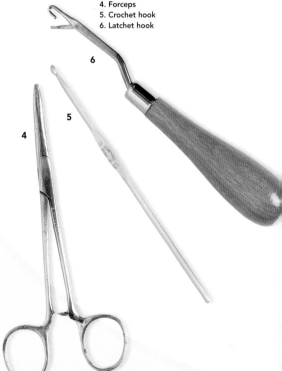

STIFFENING THE ELEMENT

If you don't wish to use any equipment for ply-split darning, a small amount of tape can be useful.

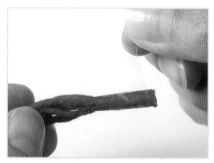

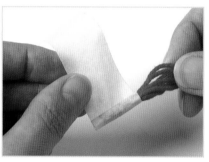

Wrapping a piece of sticky tape over the end of the weft element can help to stiffen it as if it were the end of a shoelace.

Alternatively use a piece of masking tape to stiffen the weft element.

USING A NEEDLE

If you wish to use a tool to assist in the process, a large bodkin or needle can be used to draw the weft element through the warps (as shown).

Alternatively, a latchet hook or forceps can be put through the ply and used to grasp the weft, pulling it through the warps.

TIP
If using a needle, take care that it does not pierce the plies, but goes neatly between them.

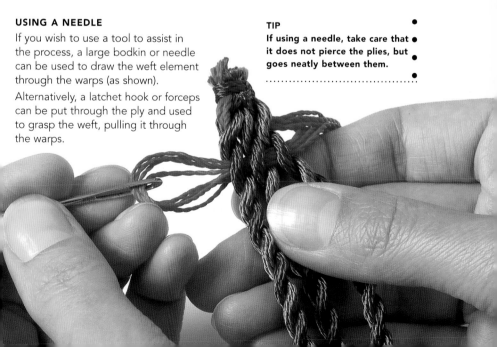

PLY-SPLIT DARNING: TWO CORDS

This technique requires a little preparation before the ply-splitting can begin. Here, the two cords used for the warps are both two-ply, Z-twist cords. Instructions on how to make these type of cords can be found in the Twisting section of the book. Another weft element is passed, back and forth, between the plies of each cord. As it goes from left to right it increases the slant of the plies. When it is passing from right to left, the slant is decreased.

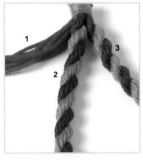

1 Join all of the elements together and arrange them in order so that Element 1 is on the left and Element 3 is on the right.

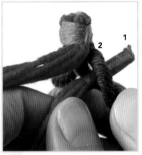

2 Start with the first slanting stitch of Element 2. Open a space between the plies of Element 2 and take Element 1 through the space, from left to right.

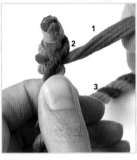

3 Pull Element 1 until it is fully drawn through Element 2.

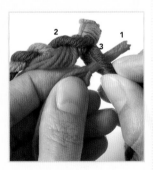

4 Open a space in the first slanting stitch of Element 3. Take Element 1 through the space from left to right.

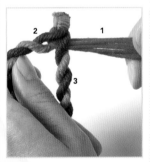

5 Pull Element 1 until it is fully drawn through Element 3.

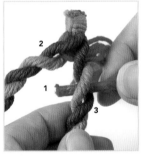

6 Now open a space in the next slanting stitch on Element 3. Take Element 1 through the space from right to left. There should be a half twist left in the cord, between the two passings of Element 1.

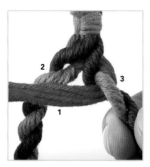

7 Pull Element 1 until it is fully drawn through Element 3.

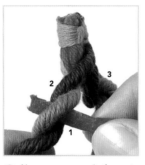

8 Now open a space in the next slanting stitch on Element 2. Take Element 1 through the space from right to left. There should be a half twist left in the cord, between the two passings of Element 1.

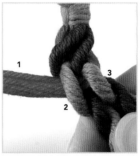

9 Pull Element 1 until it is fully drawn through Element 2.

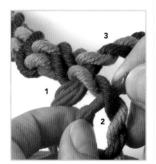

10 Repeat Steps 2 to 9, always using the next stitch below, so that a half twist is left in the cord between each passing of Element 1.

TIP
If you untwist the cord a little, a space will open up between the plies.

A partially worked sample of two cord ply-splitting.

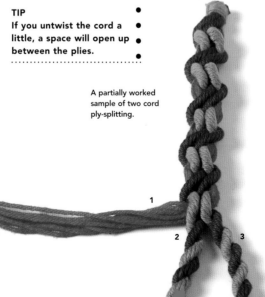

PLY-SPLIT DARNING: THREE CORDS

This can be worked in the same way as the two-cord version, with extra steps to introduce the fourth element on the right. However, these instructions show how a bodkin is used to draw the weft through the warp cords. It is not necessary to use a tool such as this, but it does speed up the process.

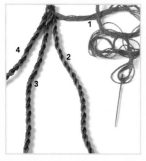

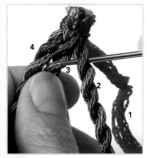

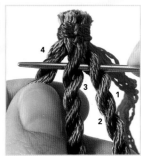

1 Thread Element 1 onto a bodkin, then join all of the elements together. Arrange them so that Element 1 starts on the right and Elements 2 to 4 are in order from right to left.

2 Start with the first slanting stitch of Element 2. Insert the bodkin between the two plies from right to left.

3 Open a space in the first slanting stitch of Element 3. Insert the bodkin between the two plies from right to left.

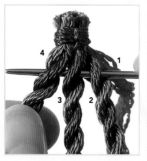

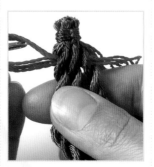

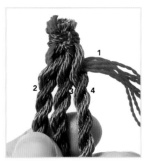

4 Open a space in the first slanting stitch of Element 4. Insert the bodkin between the two plies from right to left.

5 Pull the bodkin through the three warp elements, drawing Element 1 with it. Keep pulling Element 1 until it is fully drawn through the other elements

6 Turn the work over so that Element 1 is back on the right-hand side.

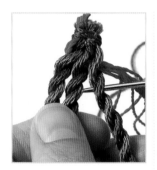

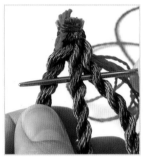

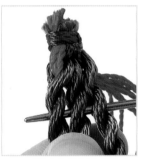

7　Open a space in the next slanting stitch on Element 4 and insert the bodkin from right to left. There should be a half twist left in the cord, between the previous passing of Element 1 and the bodkin.

8　Now open a space in the next slanting stitch on Element 3, and insert the bodkin into this space, from right to left.

9　Pull Element 1 until it is fully drawn through Element 2.

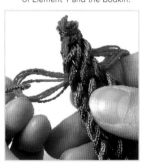

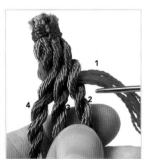

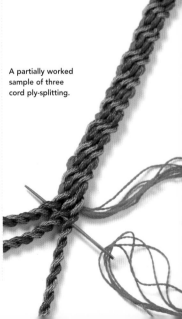

10　Pull the bodkin through the three warp elements, drawing Element 1 with it.

11　Turn the work over so that Element 1 is back on the right-hand side. Make sure that it is pulled firmly through all of the other elements. Repeat Steps 2 to 10, always using the next stitch below, so that a half twist is left in the cord between each passing of Element 1.

A partially worked sample of three cord ply-splitting.

Working with Beads

Threads and beads make wonderful combinations. The hard, shiny, lustrous quality of the beads contrast against the soft, textural qualities of thread, providing unique design possibilities. The selection of bead types is enormous, as is the range of threads, so there are endless possibilities for combining the two.

USING STRINGS OF BEADS

Beads can be bought prethreaded on strings. These can be wonderful labor-saving items, but care must be taken to ensure that the thread is strong enough for the intended purpose. Although strings are flexible, they are not suitable for intensive bending. All of the samples shown in this book require manipulation in some manner. This puts a strain on the thread—there is nothing worse than your beautiful work suddenly exploding. Always thread your beads onto a strong thread. You can either use a special beading thread or a strong sewing thread; these can also be waxed for further protection. The size of the bead holes often dictates which thread you can use. If possible, use several strands rather than a single one to increase the strength. Try out different-size beading needles and quantities of thread.

As the strings are manipulated, the beads are forced apart, causing pressure to build up. At the start of the work, the beads are forced toward the end of the string and you need to release some tension. This is why it is best to put the beads onto threads that are longer than the actual quantity of beads. As a rough guide use 47–51 in (120–130 cm) of thread for 39 in (100 cm) length of beads. This allows you to ease the beads gradually down the thread, releasing some of the tension. Some threads are naturally more elastic than others so the take-up rate will vary.

USING A BEAD SPINNER

You can use a bead spinner to speed up the process of adding beads onto your thread.

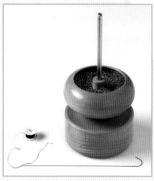

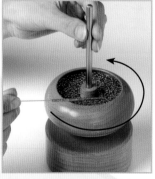

TIP
It is always a good idea to overestimate the string length required, so that you are not trying to fiddle around with short lengths at the end of your work.

The beads are placed in a bowl that rotates around the spindle.

As the spindle is twisted the bowl of beads spins around forcing the beads up the needle.

TO MAKE A STRING OF BEADS

The example shown here is preparation for making a string of size 8°
rocaille beads, 12 in (31 cm) in length.

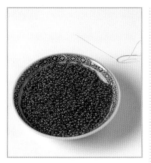

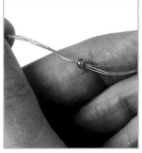

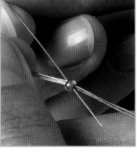

1 Fold two strands of beading
thread, each 1 yard (1 meter) in
length, in half, to create a half-
yard (50 cm) length of four
parallel strands. Thread two
strands through the beading
needle so that the needle sits
in the center of the length.

2 Add one bead and position it
along the strands so that it sits
near to the end, away from
the needle.

3 Take the needle back through
the bead in the same direction
as the first time.

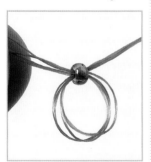

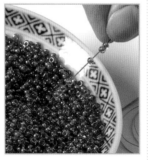

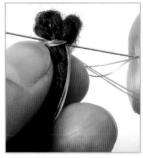

4 Tighten the thread so that the
bead stays in position. This will
act as a stopper bead,
preventing the other beads
from sliding off the thread. It
can be gently eased along the
thread when the tension
needs releasing.

5 Add the required length of
beads (12 in [31 cm]) onto the
rest of the thread. You can
either add the beads
individually, or you can try
scooping them up out of a
shallow bowl.

6 Use the needle to stitch the
strands into the beginning of
the other (textile) elements.
(Note that the beaded samples
on pages 169 and 227 are
made from just strings of
beads, so knot the threads
to secure.)

WORKING WITH STRINGS OF BEADS: TWISTING

Here, it is the thread inside the beads that twists, rather than the beads themselves. As usual, the beads need to be strung onto a thread that is longer than the required length of beads. For this method, the thread must also have plenty of room to move inside the bead hole. As the thread is twisted, it becomes shorter and fatter, so an allowance for this must be made. There is no exact formula for this, as all beads have different-size holes. However, take care not to add any small-holed beads onto the string.

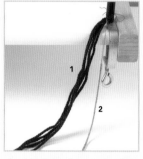

1 Join all the elements together and attach to a fixed point.

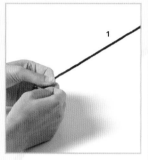

2 Twist Element 1 and secure it to prevent the twist from unraveling.

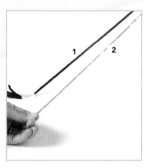

3 Now take Element 2 (the string of beads) and remove the stopper bead from the end of the string. Carefully spread the rest of the beads along the whole length of the thread.

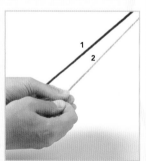

4 Add the twist to the strands of the string of beads, rather than to the beads. When sufficient twist has been added, push all the beads up together toward the fixed point.

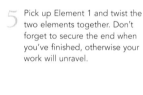

5 Pick up Element 1 and twist the two elements together. Don't forget to secure the end when you've finished, otherwise your work will unravel.

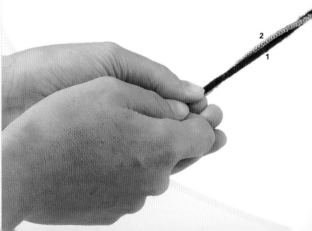

WORKING WITH STRINGS OF BEADS: OTHER TECHNIQUES

Strings of beads have also been used in all the other sections (knotting, interlooping, weaving, braiding, and ply-split darning). However, here the beads play an active part in the process. The bead stopper is left in place to keep the whole string as a firm working unit. Strings of beads are not as flexible as ordinary threads, so you will have to work a little looser, moving the strings in gentle curves, rather than tight bends.

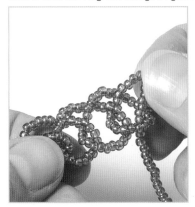

1 Here, a string of beads is being interlooped. As the strings are manipulated, the beads are forced apart, building up the pressure on the thread.

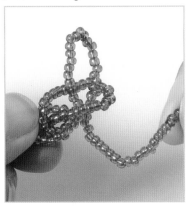

2 Here, the string is too tight. Release the pressure by gently easing the stopper bead down the string. Try to do this little and often, in order to keep the tension of the whole piece looking even.

TIP
Try putting a pin into the stopper bead to help you ease it down gradually.

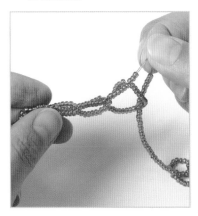

3 Be careful not to ease the stopper bead down too far. As you can see from the example here, this makes the work too loose, with bits of the thread showing between the beads.

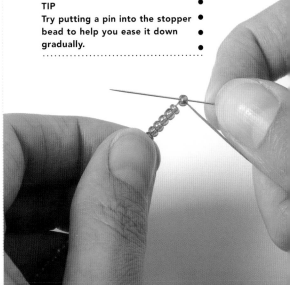

ADDING BEADS BEFORE THE WORKING PROCESS: SINGLES

Beads can be added onto the elements before work begins. The size of the bead hole must be compatible with the size of the element you are trying to thread it onto. Unfortunately, the size of the holes can vary considerably, even within the same packet. If the beads will not fit, try making the sample with finer threads, or fewer strands. A needle can be used to help thread the bead. However, the bead will not always fit over both the needle eye and the element at the same time. Using a leader thread will resolve this problem. The sample in the following steps is on page 151.

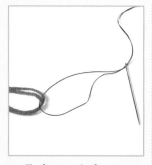

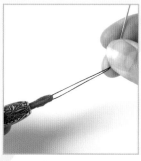

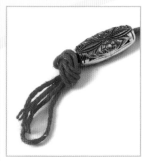

1 The four strands of cotton are created by folding two strands in half. Thread a fine leader thread through the loops of the element and take both ends through the eye of a needle.

2 Thread the bead over the needle, onto the leader thread, then onto the element.

3 Put an overhand knot in the end of the element to stop the beads from falling off the end. Once the beads have been added to the elements, work can commence.

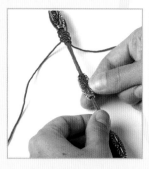

4 Keep the beads at the lower end of the element until they are required. To introduce a bead, you will need to push a single bead up the element until it sits close against the work. As normal working practices resume, it will do so below the bead.

TIP
A small blob of glue on the end of the element strengthens it, making it easier to push the beads onto. Take time to make sure that the tension and spacing are even, so that the bead sits snugly in the work.

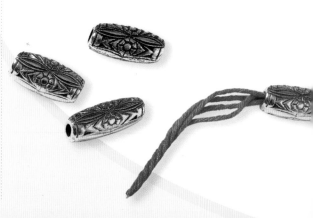

ADDING BEADS BEFORE THE WORKING PROCESS: MULTIPLE BEADS

In these samples the beads are introduced into the work as a set of beads, rather than individually. This causes the beaded element to protrude slightly, so extra care must be taken when resuming your work. Allow the beads to be forced outward away from the work, forming a slight bow shape. Take care that they don't slip into the work at the start, but remain outside of the other elements.

ADDING BEADS DURING THE WORKING PROCESS

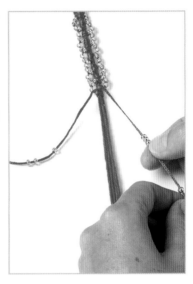

Alternatively, beads can be added during the working practice like the beaded samples on pages 143, 187, and 243. It is impossible to produce the sample on page 187 by adding the beads at any other stage since all of the elements must pass through the bead after they have worked together to produce some weaving. The other samples could have the beads added onto the elements before work begins. Then as work progresses they could be introduced in the appropriate place by pushing the beads up against the work (as shown opposite). However, beads can inhibit working practices, particularly with the ply-split darning in the sample on page 243. Here the beads would have to be pushed between the plies of the other elements. Therefore, it is easier to add the beads onto the elements only when they are required.

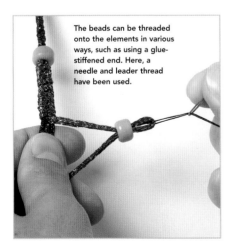

The beads can be threaded onto the elements in various ways, such as using a glue-stiffened end. Here, a needle and leader thread have been used.

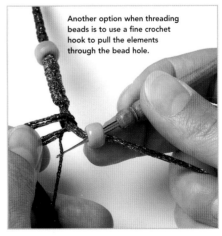

Another option when threading beads is to use a fine crochet hook to pull the elements through the bead hole.

Beginnings and ends

Many of the samples shown in this book will unravel if the ends are not secured. It is normal to make a temporary tie (with thread or even sticky tape) before taking the time to make a more permanent fixing. Both the beginning and the end of your narrow ware can be finished off in an elegant way. However, some effects, such as the smooth start, can only be made on the beginning of some samples.

WHIPPING

This is a basic way of securing a narrow ware. It can be made anywhere along the length of the sample, so you can create exactly the length you require. You can even make two whippings in the center of the sample and cut between them, thus making two sections. Ideally, use a strand of the same type found in the sample, so that the whipping matches the rest of the work. Here a contrasting color has been used to highlight the whipping.

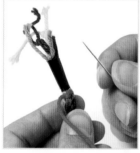 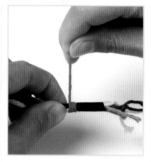 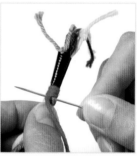

1 Secure the whipping strand into the sample by making a couple of stitches on top of each other. Note the temporary tie is still holding the sample secure while work is in progress.

2 Wind the whipping strand around the sample. To make a neat start, you can cover the stitches used to secure the strand. A better result can be achieved by keeping the strand taut and lying parallel.

3 Secure the end of the strand back into the sample with a couple more stitches on top of each other and above the whipping.

4 To make the whipping extra secure and prevent it from slipping down the sample, you can make another stitch over the whipping, before stitching back into the sample. Trim away the loose ends.

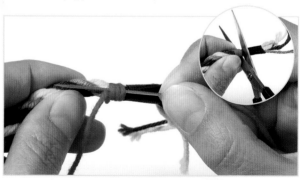

SIMPLE TASSEL

Rather than trim away the loose ends, they can be used to make a simple tassel.

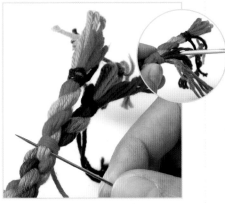

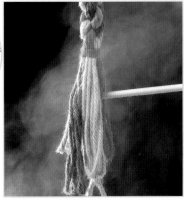

1 Make a whipping. Remove the temporary tie and unravel any stitches below the whipping. The end of a knitting needle can help ease out the strands.

2 Gently steam the strands to straighten them. Take care not to scald your fingers. Again, a chopstick or knitting needle can be useful for easing out the threads.

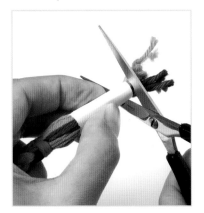

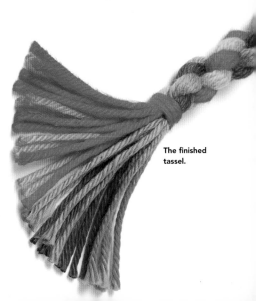

The finished tassel.

4 Roll a small piece of paper around the strands and use this as a guide to cut the ends of the tassel evenly.

ADDITIONAL TASSEL

Sometimes the strands used in the sample are not sufficient for making a feature of the tassel. In this case, additional strands can be used. They can be of the same type used in the sample, or they can even be something completely different! Different threads have different properties and some drape better than others. It is worth experimenting with a range of options to see which effect you feel is right for your project. Here, a tassel of glitter thread is being added to the braided sample on page 217.

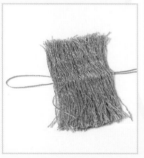

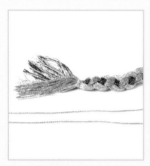

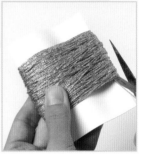

1. Prepare a thread for tying the tassel. Here a piece of pearl cotton of about 16 in (41 cm) in length has been folded in half and is laid out ready for the tassel. Prepare the sample by whipping the end.

2. Cut a piece of card a little deeper than you wish the tassel to be. Pinch the end of the glitter thread and wind it around the card.

3. The more thread is wound around the card the fuller the final tassel will be. Here the strand is taken around the card 200 times. Cut the strands along the bottom edge of the card.

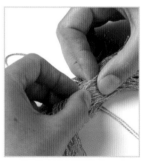

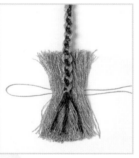

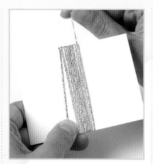

4. Carefully lay the tassel strands over the thread on the table so that the thread lies across the center.

5. Lay the sample on top of the tassel strands so that it lies parallel and the whipping is resting just below the tying thread.

6. Roll the tassel strands around the sample.

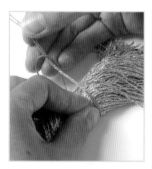

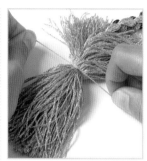

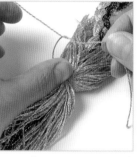

7 Tie the tassel strands with the pearl cotton by taking both of the ends through the loop (forming a lark's head knot).

8 Take the ends in opposite directions right around the tassel.

9 Tie the ends together in a reef knot.

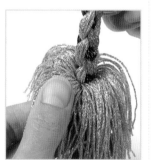

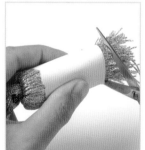

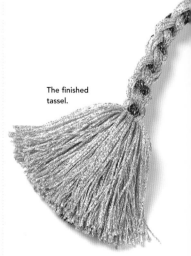

10 Lift the sample and shake down the tassel strands.

11 Roll a small piece of paper around the strands and use this as a guide to cut the ends of the tassel evenly.

The finished tassel.

SMOOTH STARTS

A smooth start gives a clean, unfussy line on one end of the sample and is possible on some, but not all, of the samples. The strands need to start in loops, so it all depends on numbers. Two examples are shown, each dealing with different aspects of creating loops. Other examples will need modifying slightly, but the principle will be the same. Unfortunately, it is not possible to achieve the same effect on the other end of the sample as there will always be the ends of the strands to contend with.

EVEN ELEMENTS

This shows a smooth start for the braided sample on page 213. Here, each of the four elements are made up of a single strand. Although the element is made from an odd numbered strand, loops can be made by connecting the even number of elements together.

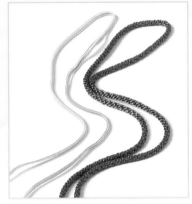

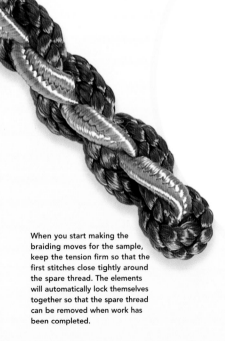

1 Cut one strand of lacing cord, twice the required length for one element. Cut a strand of Russia braid, twice the required length for one element.

When you start making the braiding moves for the sample, keep the tension firm so that the first stitches close tightly around the spare thread. The elements will automatically lock themselves together so that the spare thread can be removed when work has been completed.

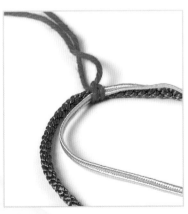

2 Use a piece of thread to tie the lengths together at the center. Fold the strands in half—each half provides the strand for one element. The spare thread can be used to attach the elements to a fixed point.

EVEN STRANDS

This shows a smooth start for the twisted sample on page 123. Here, the two elements are odd as they are of different colors. However, they each consist of an even number of strands from which the loops can be made, although care must be taken to ensure they connect to each other.

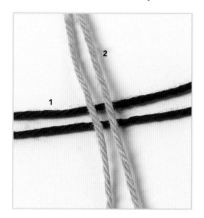

1 Cut two strands of cotton (1), twice the required length for one element. Cut two strands of cotton (2), twice the required length for another element. Lay as shown.

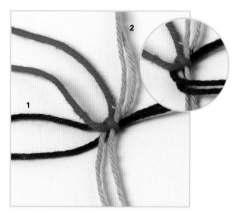

2 Tie the centers together with a piece of spare thread. Bring one half of 1 over 2, so that it becomes the element of four strands.

The elements will automatically lock themselves together so that the spare thread can be removed when work has been completed.

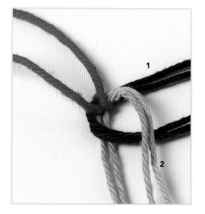

3 Now bring the ends of the number 2 strands together to make the other element of four strands. Use the spare thread to attach the work to a fixed point.

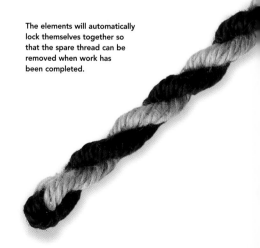

LOOPED STARTS

This is another feature that can only be achieved on some samples, and again it requires an even numbers of elements or strands. However, it is a very useful start because it produces a strong neat loop that is an integral part of the finished sample. Unfortunately, it is not possible to achieve a similar effect on the other end of the sample. The example shown makes a looped start on the sample on page 159. Any of the strands could be used to make the covering knots, so you can decide what color or texture you wish to make the loop. Don't forget to add extra length to allow for the take-up of the loop.

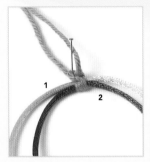

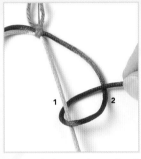

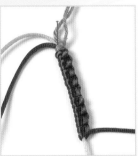

1. Cut a strand of rattail (1), twice the required length for one element, plus 2 in (5 cm)—the diameter of the loop. Cut another strand (2) twice the required length, plus 18 in (46 cm) for the take-up of the knotting. Use a piece of spare thread to tie the two strands together near the midway point.

2. Use the longest Element 2 and make a series of opposite half hitches (see page 34, Right Hand Over, Right Hand Under) over the top of the longest Element 1.

3. Continue until 2 in (5 cm) of Element 1 have been covered.

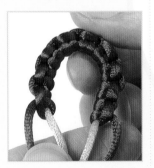

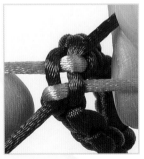

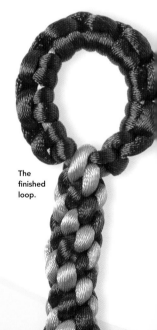

The finished loop.

4. Remove the spare thread and fold the half hitches, bringing the start and end of them together to form the loop.

5. Start the sample, taking care to tension the first few stitches so that they sit snugly against the loop.

BELL CAPS

Covering the ends of a sample with a bell cap produces a smooth neat finish, as well as providing a means of attaching jewelry fittings. A bell cap can be connected to a clasp to make a bracelet or necklace, or it can be joined to an earring wire. There are many types of bell caps, from mass-produced, pronged caps, to handmade designs such as the one shown in this example. It is critical that the size of the bell cap is compatible to the sample, so it is worth checking the fit before applying the glue.

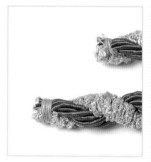

1 Whip the end of the sample and trim away the ends of the elements.

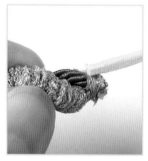

2 Apply a small amount of two-part epoxy adhesive over the whipping.

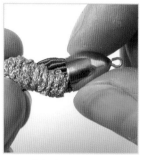

3 Push the bell cap onto the whipped end and leave to dry.

Both the start and finish of the narrow ware have been fitted with bell caps. They have then been attached to a necklace clasp.

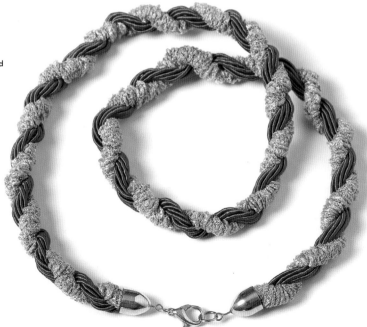

Using Narrow Wares

Narrow wares can be put to many uses, either as a finishing touch to other projects, or as items in their own right. The advantage of making your own narrow wares is that you can alter the size, shape, texture, and color of the work so that it is ideally suited for your purpose.

Adding trims onto textiles is a popular way of using narrow wares. Examples can be found all over the world and throughout history. There are many different ways of attaching the trims and a couple are explored here. They can be stitched down using a needle and thread. Ideally, the thread should be a strand of the same type used in the narrow ware. However, this is not always possible. Sometimes the strands used in the narrow ware are too fragile, or too thick, to use for stitching. If this is the case, you will have to find an appropriate alternative for stitching down your work.

STARTING AND FINISHING

The question of what to do with the ends of a trim really depends on the project. Here are two solutions for hiding the ends. The ends of the braid have been whipped in advance, which prevents the work from unraveling.

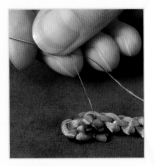

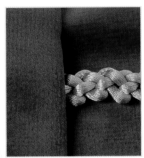

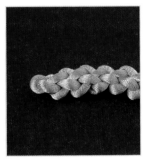

1 Fold over the end of the narrow ware so that it is tucked under the braid and hidden from view.

2 The end has been pushed into a gap in the seam, so it is hidden behind the fabric.

Another neat option is to use a smooth start, so that there are no loose strand ends to hide. Of course, this can only be used at the beginning of the trim, so an alternative will be needed for the other end.

COUCHING

Trims can be couched down onto fabric to hide seams or to form borders. They can also be used to create surface designs. Better results can be achieved if the fabric is stretched and supported by a frame.

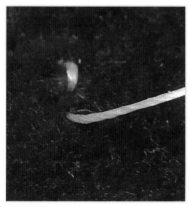

1 Secure the couching thread into the fabric with a couple of stitches on top of each other.

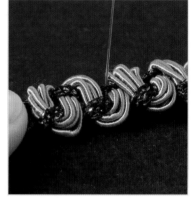

2 Lay the narrow ware onto the fabric. If you are working complex designs, it may help to baste it in place before making the final couching stitches.

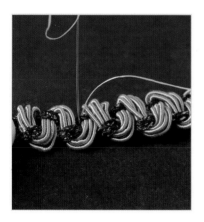

3 Take the needle down through the bottom of a stitch in the narrow ware. Make sure that the couching thread follows the line of this stitch.

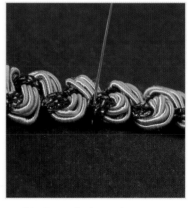

4 Take the needle along to the next narrow ware stitch and repeat the process.

EDGING

Covering the edge of a fabric seam, such as for a cushion trim, is a lovely way of framing a project. Working with a matching color would make the stitching almost invisible.

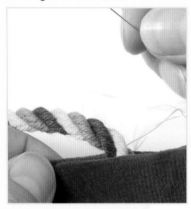

1 The start of the sample has been taken inside the seam to hide the end. The thread has been secured with a couple of stitches on top of each other.

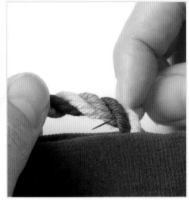

2 Take the needle from the back to the front, through the base of the cord.

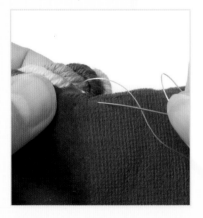

3 Take the needle into the fabric and along the inside of the seam, for a short distance. Bring it out to the back of the seam. Repeat Steps 2 and 3.

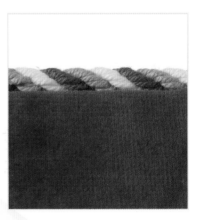

The finished edging.

BASIC CLOSURE

Narrow wares can be used to connect things together, such as ties on clothing, or closures for bags or boxes. The join can be as simple as tying two sections together in a bow. Or it can be more sophisticated like the loop and knot join. These can be used to join two separate sections together, an idea that would make attractive froggings on a jacket. Or, it can be used to join the beginning and end of one sample, making a perfect link for a necklace.

TIES

Here a connection is made with two sections of cord. Both sections have smooth starts and are finished with a simple tassel. The first inch (2.5 cm) of each section is couched down onto the fabric. The end parts are loose and can be used to make a bow or reef knot.

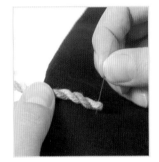

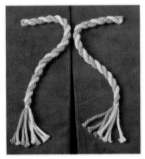

BASIC LOOP AND BUTTON

Here, a 6 in (15 cm) length of braid is used. Both ends have been finished with a simple tassel. Note that the measurements may need to be altered, depending on the diameter of the buttons.

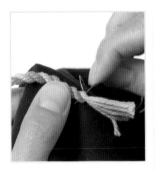

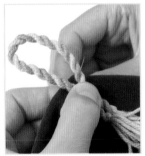

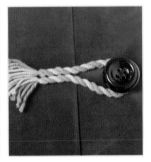

1 Start the braid 1 in (2.5 cm) away from the edge and couch it down until it reaches the edge.

2 Turn the braid to form a loop out away from the edge. Couch down the end of the braid so that it sits parallel to the start.

3 Use the loop to slip over a button.

LOOP AND KNOT

Here, one half of the join is a looped start, which is described on page 100. The other half of the join is a knot. There are many options, such as a Chinese ball knot. This double overhand knot is simple, but effective.

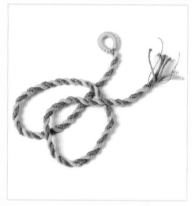

1 Prepare a sample with a looped start.

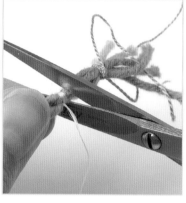

2 Whip the end of the sample. Trim away all the loose ends except for the one used to make the whipping.

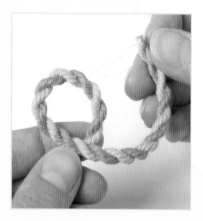

3 Make a loop toward the end of the sample.

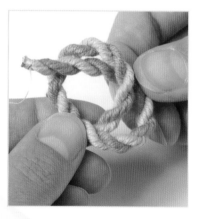

4 Take the end of the sample up through the loop.

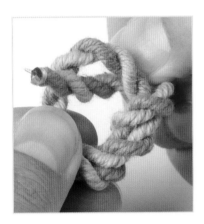

5 Take the end around the outside of the loop and back up into the loop.

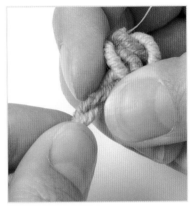

6 Tighten the knot to the end of the sample.

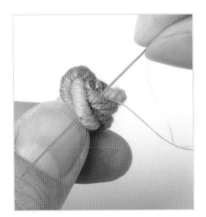

7 For extra security, use the strand from the whipping to stitch the end of the sample down against itself at the base of the knot.

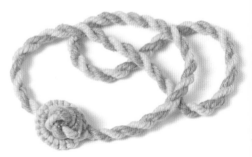

8 Use this knot to slip through the loop.

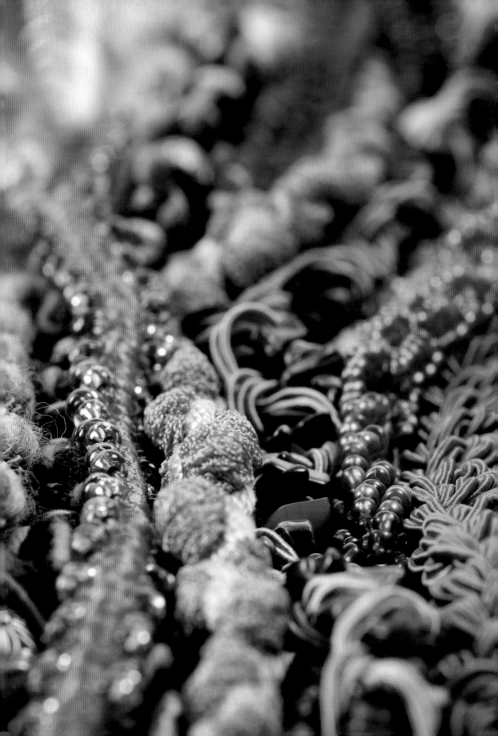

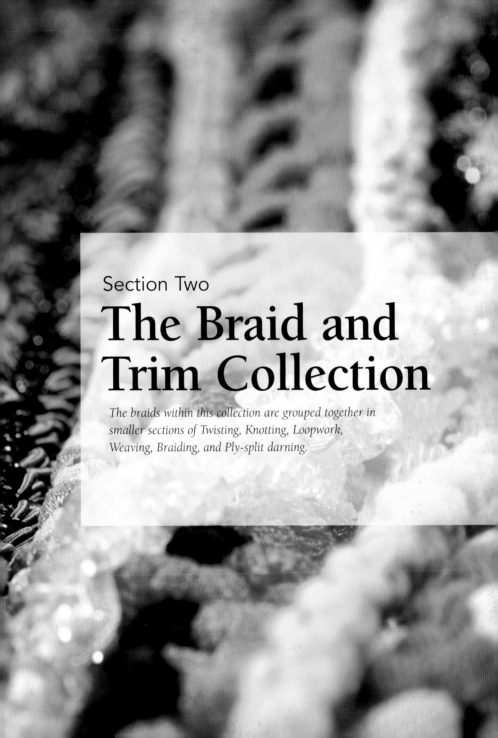

Section Two

The Braid and Trim Collection

The braids within this collection are grouped together in smaller sections of Twisting, Knotting, Loopwork, Weaving, Braiding, and Ply-split darning.

BRAID AND TRIM SELECTOR

All of the braids featured in the book appear on the following pages. Just pick the one you'd like to make and turn to the page number for more information.

TWISTING

| Page 122 | Page 124 | Page 126 | Page 128 | Page 130 | Page 132 |

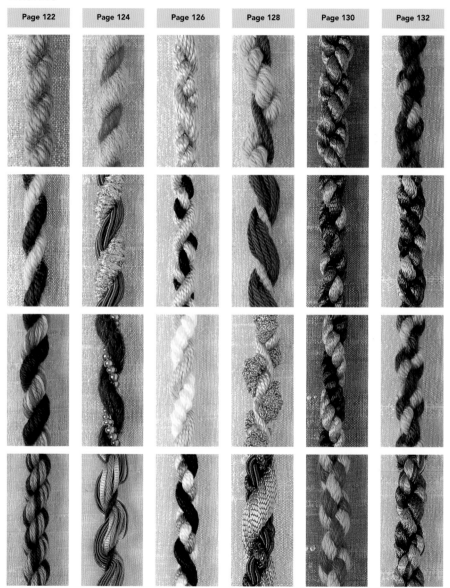

KNOTTING

Page 134	Page 136	Page 138	Page 142	Page 144	Page 146

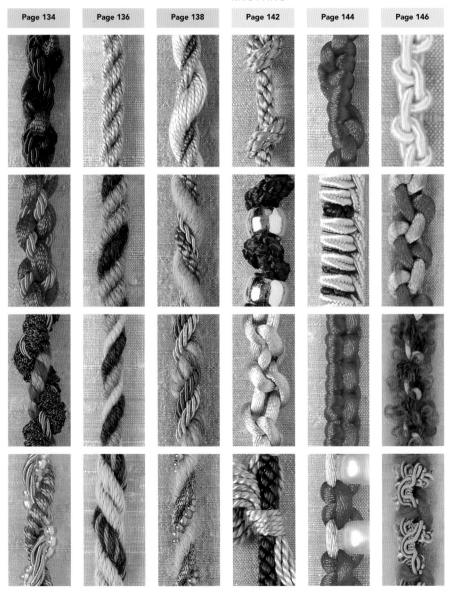

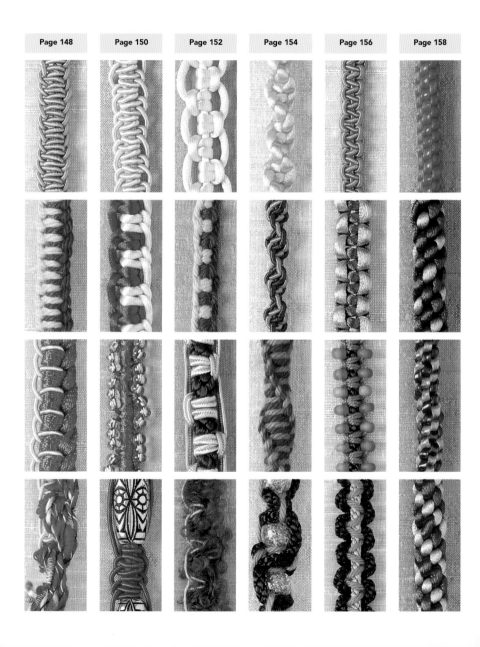

| Page 148 | Page 150 | Page 152 | Page 154 | Page 156 | Page 158 |

LOOPWORK

| Page 160 | Page 162 | Page 164 | Page 168 | Page 170 | Page 172 |

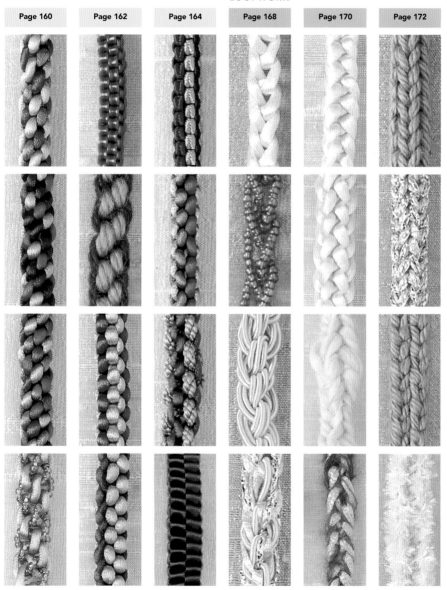

WEAVING

Page 174	Page 176	Page 178	Page 182	Page 184	Page 186

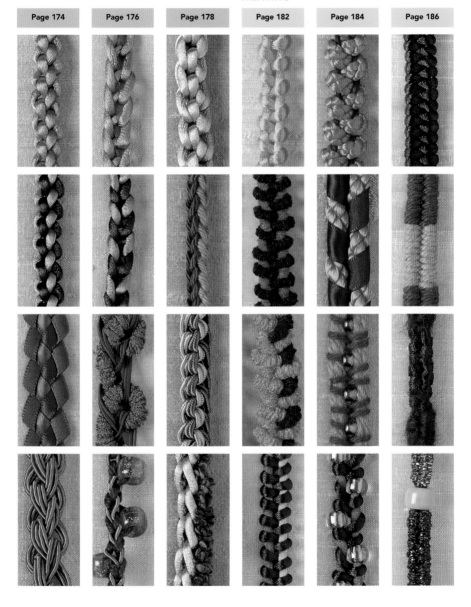

BRAIDING

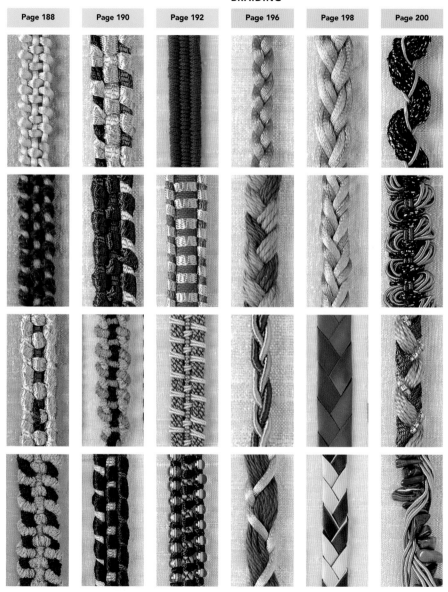

| Page 188 | Page 190 | Page 192 | Page 196 | Page 198 | Page 200 |

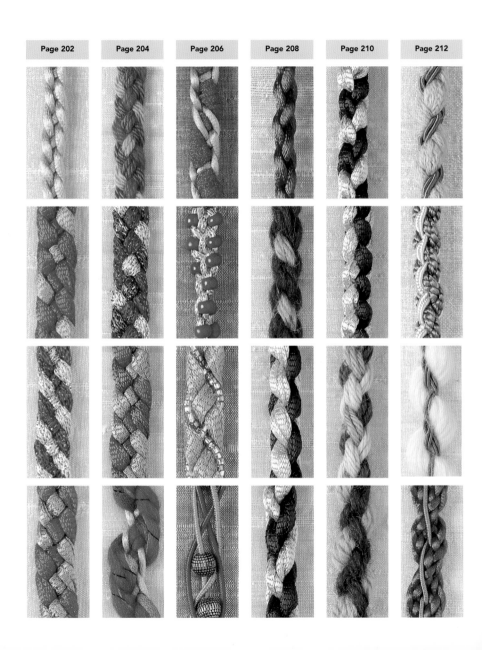

Page 202   Page 204   Page 206   Page 208   Page 210   Page 212

| Page 214 | Page 216 | Page 218 | Page 220 | Page 222 | Page 224 |

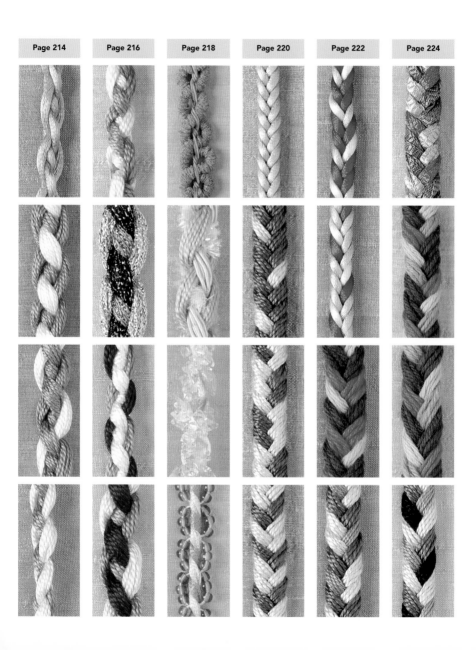

PLY-SPLIT DARNING

Page 226	Page 228	Page 230	Page 232	Page 234	Page 238

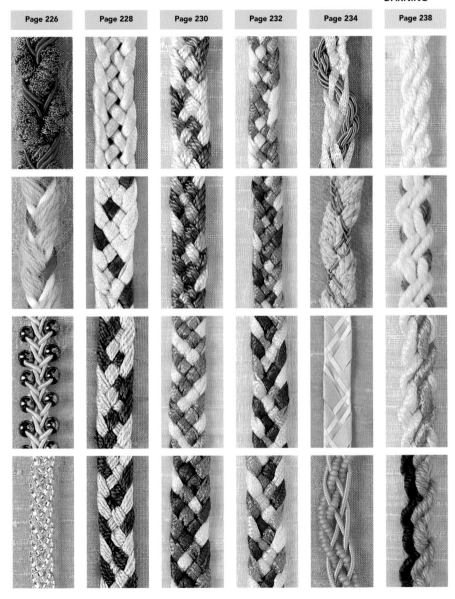

Page 240	Page 242	Page 244	Page 246	Page 248	Page 250

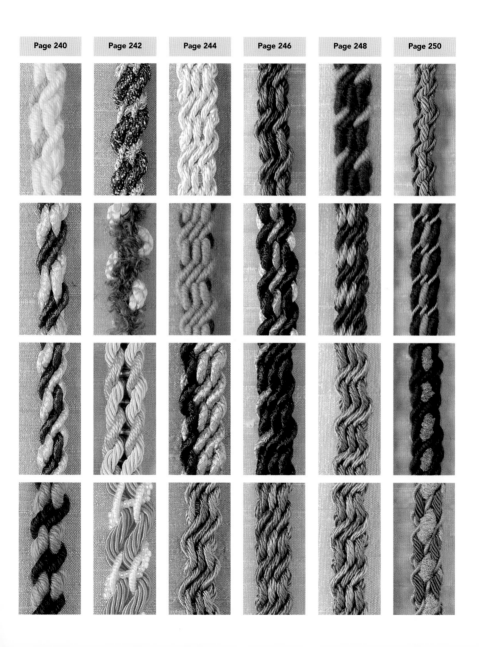

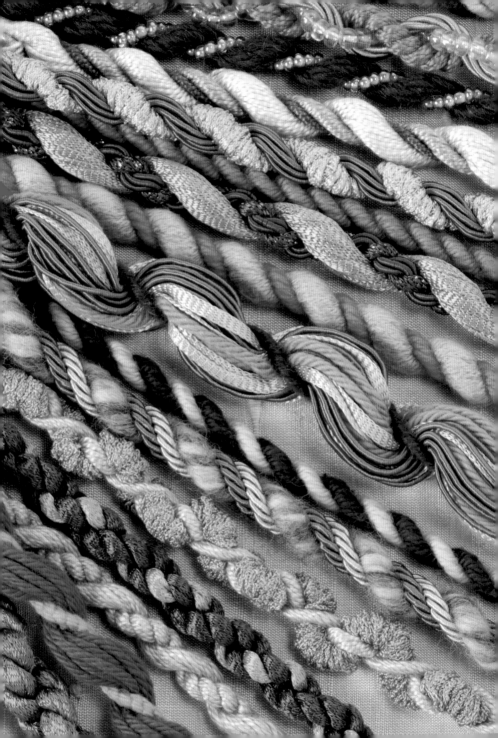

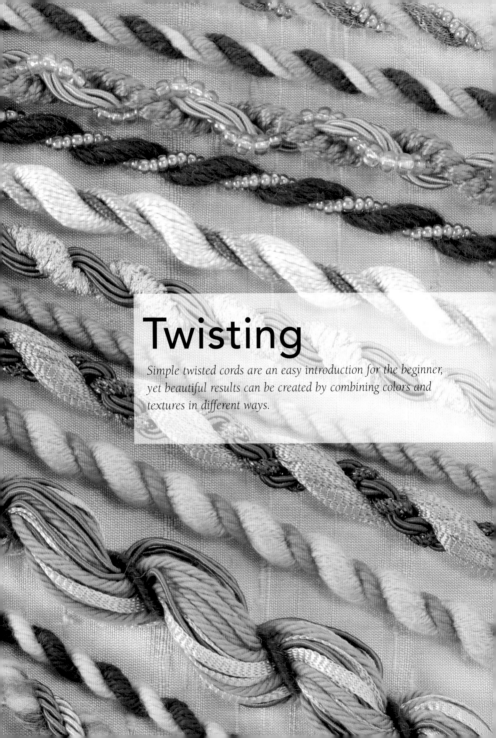

Twisting

Simple twisted cords are an easy introduction for the beginner, yet beautiful results can be created by combining colors and textures in different ways.

Two-ply

A two-ply cord is made from twisting two elements together. Although it is a basic structure, there are many possibilities for combining color and texture.

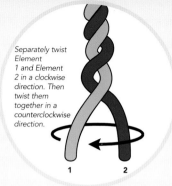

Separately twist Element 1 and Element 2 in a clockwise direction. Then twist them together in a counterclockwise direction.

1   **2**

PLAIN

Easy rating ✔

Materials

Element 1 = 16 in (41 cm) = 4 strands of mauve Double Top cotton

Element 2 = 16 in (41 cm) = 4 strands of mauve Double Top cotton

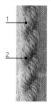

Method

Separately twist Element 1 and Element 2 in a clockwise direction. Then twist them together in a counterclockwise direction (see page 22).

TWO COLORS

Easy rating ✔

Materials

Element 1 = 16 in (41 cm) = 4 strands of purple Double Top cotton

Element 2 = 16 in (41 cm) = 4 strands of lilac Double Top cotton

Method

Separately twist Element 1 and Element 2 in a clockwise direction. Then twist them together in a counterclockwise direction (see page 22).

PLAIN AND BLENDED

Easy rating ✔

Materials

Element 1 = 17 in (43 cm) = 18 strands of purple Double Top cotton

Element 2 = 17 in (43 cm) = 6 strands of mauve, 6 strands of lilac, and 6 strands of pink Double Top cotton

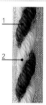

Method

Separately twist Element 1 and Element 2 in a clockwise direction. Then twist them together in a counterclockwise direction (see page 22).

TWO BLENDED

Easy rating ✔

Materials

Element 1 = 17 in (43 cm) = 9 strands of mauve and 9 strands of purple Double Top cotton

Element 2 = 17 in (43 cm) = 9 strands of mauve and 9 strands of purple Double Top cotton

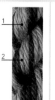

Method

Separately twist Element 1 and Element 2 in a clockwise direction. Then twist them together in a counterclockwise direction (see page 22).

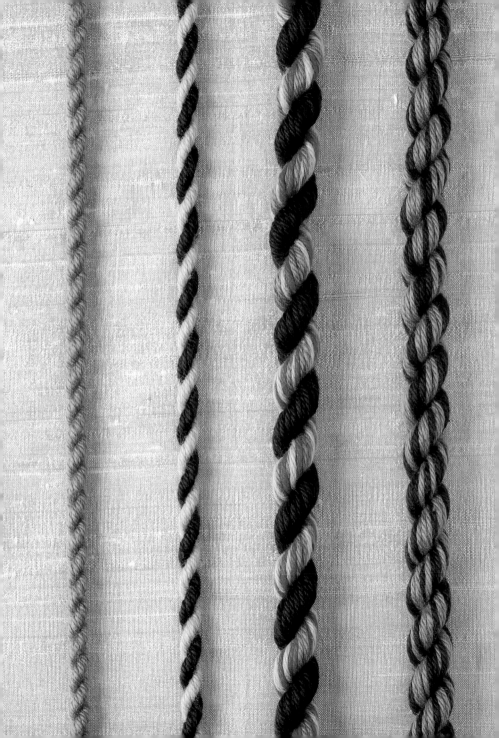

THICK AND THIN

Easy rating ✔

Materials

Element 1 = 19 in (48 cm) = 4 strands of pink Double Top cotton

Element 2 = 19 in (48 cm) = 16 strands of lilac Calmer cotton

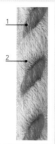

Method

Separately twist Element 1 and Element 2 in a clockwise direction. Then twist them together in a counterclockwise direction (see page 22).

GIMP AND RUCHED RIBBON

Easy rating ✔

Materials

Element 1 = 15 in (38 cm) = 8 strands of purple gimp

Element 2 = 15 in (38 cm) = 1 strand of lilac ruched knitting ribbon

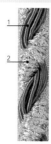

Method

Separately twist Element 1 and Element 2 in a clockwise direction. Then twist them together in a counterclockwise direction (see page 22).

WOOL AND BEADS

Easy rating ✔✔

Materials

Element 1 = 15 in (38 cm) = 4 strands of purple Chunky wool

Element 2 = 12 in (30 cm) = 1 string of size 8° lilac rocaille beads

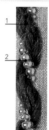

Method

Follow the instructions for Two-ply Cord (see page 22) but reverse the twist direction to make an S-twist cord. Also see page 90.

BLENDED TEXTURE

Easy rating ✔✔

Materials

Element 1 = 17 in (43 cm) = 2 strands of purple Chunky wool

Element 2 = 15 in (38 cm) = 14 strands of mauve gimp, 14 strands of lilac knitting ribbon, and 14 strands of mauve Double Top cotton

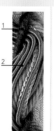

Method

Separately twist Element 1 and Element 2 in a clockwise direction. Then twist them together in a counterclockwise direction (see page 22).

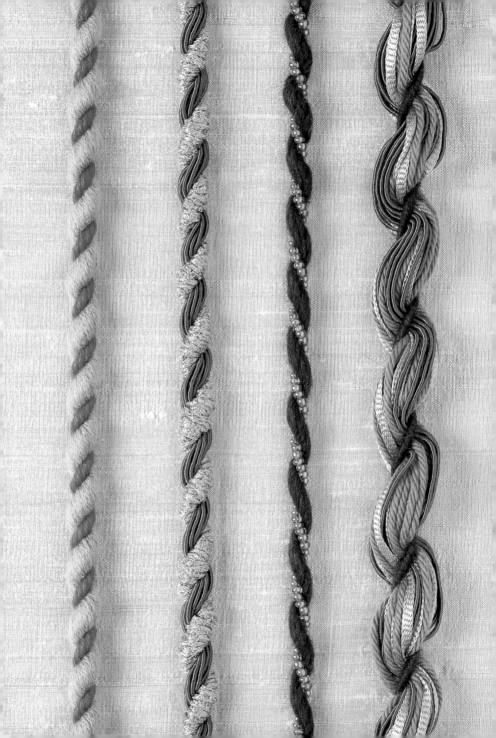

Two-ply, One-cabled

It is possible to use a premade cord as one of the elements. The following samples are made using a mixture of loose threads and one premade cord. This gives an interesting texture to the finished cord. It is important to make sure that the premade cord is retwisted in the correct direction, so that the twist is tightened rather than loosened. The results are known as retwisted, redoubled, double spun, or cabled.

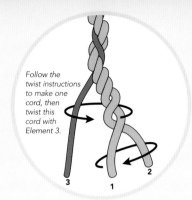

Follow the twist instructions to make one cord, then twist this cord with Element 3.

PLAIN
Easy rating ✔

Materials
Element 1 = 17 in (43 cm) = 10 strands of blue No 5 pearl cotton

Element 2 = 17 in (43 cm) = 10 strands of blue No 5 pearl cotton

Element 3 = 14 in (36 cm) = 10 strands of blue No 5 pearl cotton

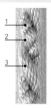

Method
Follow the instructions for Two-ply Cord (see page 22), using Elements 1 and 2. Retwist this cord with Element 3, using the instructions for Cabling with One Cord (see page 24).

TWO COLORS SPOT
Easy rating ✔

Materials
Element 1 = 17 in (43 cm) = 10 strands of navy No 5 pearl cotton

Element 2 = 17 in (43 cm) = 10 strands of blue No 5 pearl cotton

Element 3 = 14 in (36 cm) = 10 strands of blue No 5 pearl cotton

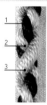

Method
Follow the instructions for Two-ply Cord (see page 22), using Elements 1 and 2, but reverse the direction of the twist to make an S-twist cord. Retwist this cord with Element 3, using the instructions for Cabling with One Cord (see page 24) but reverse the direction of the twist.

TWO COLORS STRIPE
Easy rating ✔

Materials
Element 1 = 17 in (43 cm) = 10 strands of cream No 5 pearl cotton

Element 2 = 17 in (43 cm) = 10 strands of cream No 5 pearl cotton

Element 3 = 14 in (36 cm) = 10 strands of yellow No 5 pearl cotton

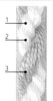

Method
Follow the instructions for Two-ply Cord (see page 22), using Elements 1 and 2, but reverse the direction of the twist to make an S-twist cord. Retwist this cord with Element 3, using the instructions for Cabling with One Cord (see page 24) but reverse the direction of the twist.

THREE COLORS
Easy rating ✔

Materials
Element 1 = 17 in (43 cm) = 10 strands of cream No 5 pearl cotton

Element 2 = 17 in (43 cm) = 10 strands of ocher No 5 pearl cotton

Element 3 = 14 in (36 cm) = 10 strands of navy No 5 pearl cotton

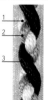

Method
Follow the instructions for Two-ply Cord (see page 22), using Elements 1 and 2. Retwist this cord with Element 3, using the instructions for Cabling with One Cord (see page 24).

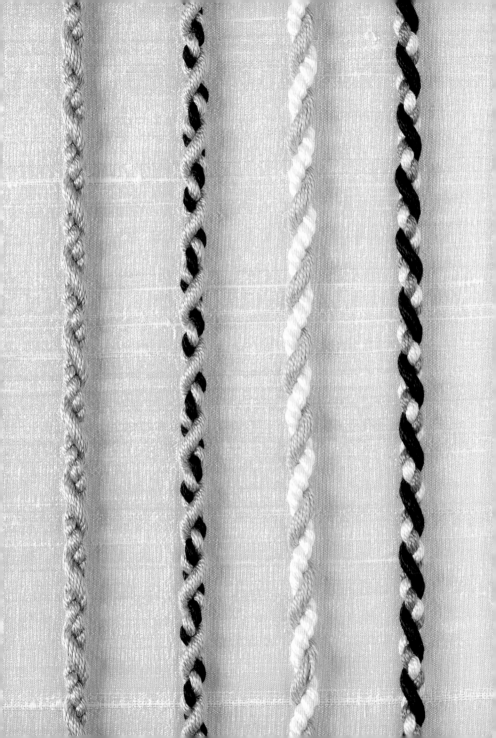

THICK CABLE

Easy rating ✔

Materials

Element 1 = 21 in (53 cm) = 8 strands of yellow Double Top cotton

Element 2 = 21 in (53 cm) = 8 strands of yellow Double Top cotton

Element 3 = 16 in (41 cm) = 4 strands of blue No 5 pearl cotton

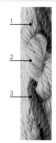

Method

Follow the instructions for Two-ply Cord (see page 22), using Elements 1 and 2. Retwist this cord with Element 3, using the instructions for Cabling with One Cord (see page 24).

THIN CABLE

Easy rating ✔

Materials

Element 1 = 17 in (43 cm) = 2 strands of yellow Double Top cotton

Element 2 = 17 in (43 cm) = 2 strands of yellow Double Top cotton

Element 3 = 15 in (38 cm) = 16 strands of blue No 5 pearl cotton

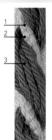

Method

Follow the instructions for Two-ply Cord (see page 22), using Elements 1 and 2. Retwist this cord with Element 3, using the instructions for Cabling with One Cord (see page 24).

RUCHED RIBBON AND COTTON

Easy rating ✔

Materials

Element 1 = 19 in (48 cm) = 1 strand of blue ruched knitting ribbon

Element 2 = 22 in (56 cm) = 10 strands of blue No 5 pearl cotton

Element 3 = 17 in (43 cm) = 10 strands of blue No 5 pearl cotton

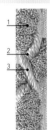

Method

Follow the instructions for Two-ply Cord (see page 22), using Elements 1 and 2. Retwist this cord with Element 3, using the instructions for Cabling with One Cord (see page 24).

THREE TEXTURES

Easy rating ✔

Materials

Element 1 = 18 in (46 cm) = 4 strands of blue gimp

Element 2 = 18 in (46 cm) = 10 strands of blue Glitter

Element 3 = 15 in (38 cm) = 20 strands of blue knitting ribbon

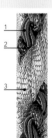

Method

Follow the instructions for Two-ply Cord (see page 22), using Elements 1 and 2, but reverse the direction of the twist to make an S-twist cord. Retwist this cord with Element 3, using the instructions for Cabling with One Cord (see page 24) but reverse the direction of the twist.

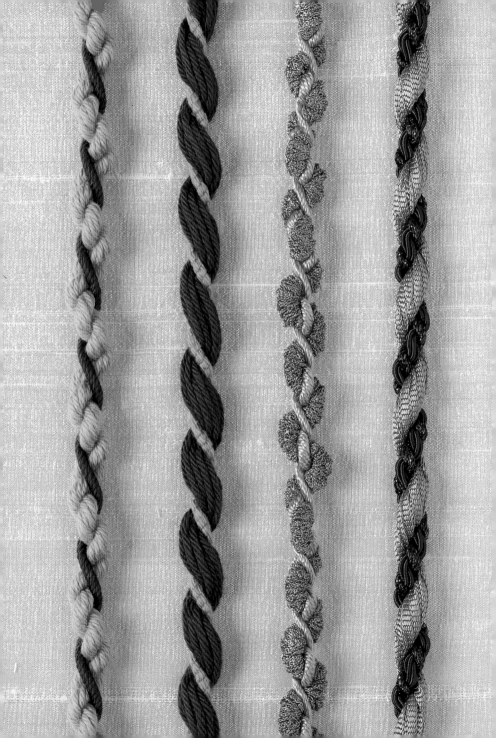

Two-ply, Two-cabled

The following samples are made from two premade cords. It is important to make sure that they are both made in the same direction—either both S- or both Z-twist.

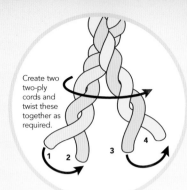

Create two two-ply cords and twist these together as required.

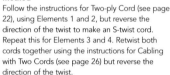

PLAIN

Easy rating ✔

Materials

Element 1 = 19 in (48 cm) = 12 strands of green knitting ribbon

Element 2 = 19 in (48 cm) = 12 strands of green knitting ribbon

Element 3 = 19 in (48 cm) = 12 strands of green knitting ribbon

Element 4 = 19 in (48 cm) = 12 strands of green knitting ribbon

Method

Follow the instructions for Two-ply Cord (see page 22), using Elements 1 and 2, but reverse the direction of the twist to make an S-twist cord. Repeat this for Elements 3 and 4. Retwist both cords together using the instructions for Cabling with Two Cords (see page 26) but reverse the direction of the twist.

TWO COLORS SPOT

Easy rating ✔

Materials

Element 1 = 19 in (48 cm) = 12 strands of yellow knitting ribbon

Element 2 = 19 in (48 cm) = 12 strands of green knitting ribbon

Element 3 = 19 in (48 cm) = 12 strands of green knitting ribbon

Element 4 = 19 in (48 cm) = 12 strands of green knitting ribbon

Method

Follow the instructions for Two-ply Cord (see page 22), using Elements 1 and 2. Repeat this for Elements 3 and 4. Retwist both cords together using the instructions for Cabling with Two Cords (see page 26).

TWO COLORS STRIPE

Easy rating ✔

Materials

Element 1 = 19 in (48 cm) = 12 strands of yellow knitting ribbon

Element 2 = 19 in (48 cm) = 12 strands of yellow knitting ribbon

Element 3 = 19 in (48 cm) = 12 strands of brown knitting ribbon

Element 4 = 19 in (48 cm) = 12 strands of brown knitting ribbon

Method

Follow the instructions for Two-ply Cord (see page 22), using Elements 1 and 2. Repeat this for Elements 3 and 4. Retwist both cords together using the instructions for Cabling with Two Cords (see page 26).

TWO COLORS DOUBLE SPOT

Easy rating ✔

Materials

Element 1 = 19 in (48 cm) = 8 strands of yellow Double Top cotton

Element 2 = 19 in (48 cm) = 8 strands of brown Double Top cotton

Element 3 = 19 in (48 cm) = 8 strands of yellow Double Top cotton

Element 4 = 19 in (48 cm) = 8 strands of brown Double Top cotton

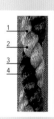
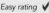

Method

Follow the instructions for Two-ply Cord (see page 22), using Elements 1 and 2, but reverse the direction of the twist to make an S-twist cord. Repeat this for Elements 3 and 4. Retwist both cords together using the instructions for Cabling with Two Cords (see page 26) but reverse the direction of the twist.

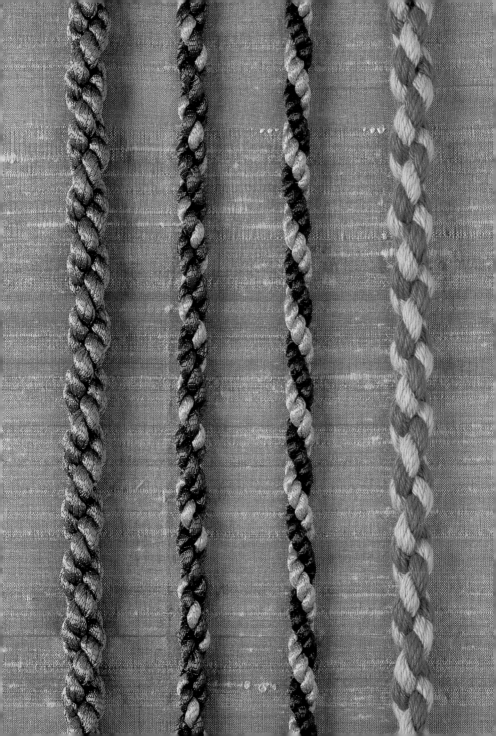

THREE COLORS SPOT AND STRIPE

Easy rating

Materials
Element 1 = 19 in (48 cm) = 4 strands of brown Double Top cotton

Element 2 = 19 in (48 cm) = 4 strands of brown Double Top cotton

Element 3 = 19 in (48 cm) = 4 strands of orange Double Top cotton

Element 4 = 19 in (48 cm) = 4 strands of green Double Top cotton

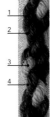

Method
Follow the instructions for Two-ply Cord (see page 22), using Elements 1 and 2. Repeat this for Elements 3 and 4. Retwist both cords together using the instructions for Cabling with Two Cords (see page 26).

THREE COLORS DOUBLE SPOT

Easy rating

Materials
Element 1 = 21 in (53 cm) = 6 strands of green knitting ribbon

Element 2 = 21 in (53 cm) = 6 strands of brown knitting ribbon

Element 3 = 21 in (53 cm) = 6 strands of yellow knitting ribbon

Element 4 = 21 in (53 cm) = 6 strands of green knitting ribbon

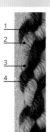

Method
Follow the instructions for Two-ply Cord (see page 22), using Elements 1 and 2, but reverse the direction of the twist to make an S-twist cord. Repeat this for Elements 3 and 4. Retwist both cords together using the instructions for Cabling with Two Cords (see page 26) but reverse the direction of the twist.

FOUR COLORS

Easy rating

Materials
Element 1 = 19 in (48 cm) = 4 strands of brown Double Top cotton

Element 2 = 19 in (48 cm) = 4 strands of orange Double Top cotton

Element 3 = 19 in (48 cm) = 4 strands of yellow Double Top cotton

Element 4 = 19 in (48 cm) = 4 strands of green Double Top cotton

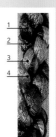

Method
Follow the instructions for Two-ply Cord (see page 22), using Elements 1 and 2. Repeat this for Elements 3 and 4. Retwist both cords together using the instructions for Cabling with Two Cords (see page 26).

TWO COLORS BLENDED

Easy rating

Materials
Element 1 = 20 in (51 cm) = 12 strands of green knitting ribbon

Element 2 = 20 in (51 cm) = 12 strands of light green knitting ribbon

Element 3 = 20 in (51 cm) = 2 strands of yellow, 2 strands of ocher, 2 strands of brown, 2 strands of orange, 2 strands of copper, 2 strands of chestnut knitting ribbon

Element 4 = 20 in (51 cm) = 2 strands of yellow, 2 strands of ocher, 2 strands of brown, 2 strands of orange, 2 strands of copper, 2 strands of chestnut knitting ribbon

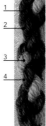

Method
Follow the instructions for Two-ply Cord (see page 22), using Elements 1 and 2, but reverse the direction of the twist to make an S-twist cord. Repeat this for Elements 3 and 4. Retwist both cords together using the instructions for Cabling with Two Cords (see page 26) but reverse the direction of the twist.

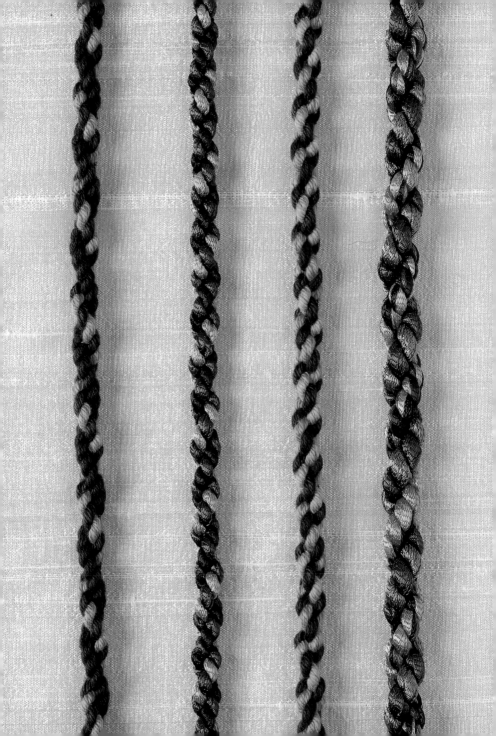

GIMP, WOOL, AND KNITTING RIBBON

Easy rating ✔

Materials

Element 1 = 19 in (48 cm) = 4 strands of green gimp

Element 2 = 19 in (48 cm) = 4 strands of green gimp

Element 3 = 19 in (48 cm) = 12 strands of green knitting ribbon

Element 4 = 19 in (48 cm) = 12 strands of green Yorkshire Tweed Aran

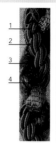

Method

Follow the instructions for Two-ply Cord (see page 22), using Elements 1 and 2. Repeat this for Elements 3 and 4. Retwist both cords together using the instructions for Cabling with Two Cords (see page 26).

GIMP AND KNITTING RIBBON

Easy rating ✔

Materials

Element 1 = 22 in (56 cm) = 4 strands of orange gimp

Element 2 = 20 in (51 cm) = 16 strands of brown knitting ribbon

Element 3 = 20 in (51 cm) = 4 strands of orange gimp

Element 4 = 20 in (51 cm) = 16 strands of brown knitting ribbon

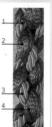

Method

Follow the instructions for Two-ply Cord (see page 22), using Elements 1 and 2. Repeat this for Elements 3 and 4. Retwist both cords together using the instructions for Cabling with Two Cords (see page 26).

RUCHED RIBBON, GIMP, AND COTTON

Easy rating ✔

Materials

Element 1 = 18 in (46 cm) = 1 strand of green ruched ribbon

Element 2 = 18 in (46 cm) = 6 strands of green gimp

Element 3 = 20 in (51 cm) = 4 strands of orange Double Top cotton

Element 4 = 20 in (51 cm) = 4 strands of brown Double Top cotton

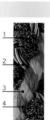

Method

Follow the instructions for Two-ply Cord (see page 22), using Elements 1 and 2, but reverse the direction of the twist to make an S-twist cord. Repeat this for Elements 3 and 4. Retwist both cords together using the instructions for Cabling with Two Cords (see page 26), but reverse the direction of the twist.

BEADS, GIMP, AND COTTON

Easy rating ✔✔

Materials

Element 1 = 15 in (38 cm) = 4 strands of ocher gimp

Element 2 = 13 in (33 cm) = 1 string of size 6° beads

Element 3 = 19 in (48 cm) = 12 strands of ocher No 5 pearl cotton

Element 4 = 19 in (48 cm) = 12 strands of ocher No 5 pearl cotton

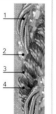

Method

Follow the instructions for Two-ply Cord (see page 22), using Elements 1 and 2, but reverse the direction of the twist to make an S-twist cord. Repeat this for Elements 3 and 4. Retwist both cords together using the instructions for Cabling with Two Cords (see page 26), but reverse the direction of the twist.

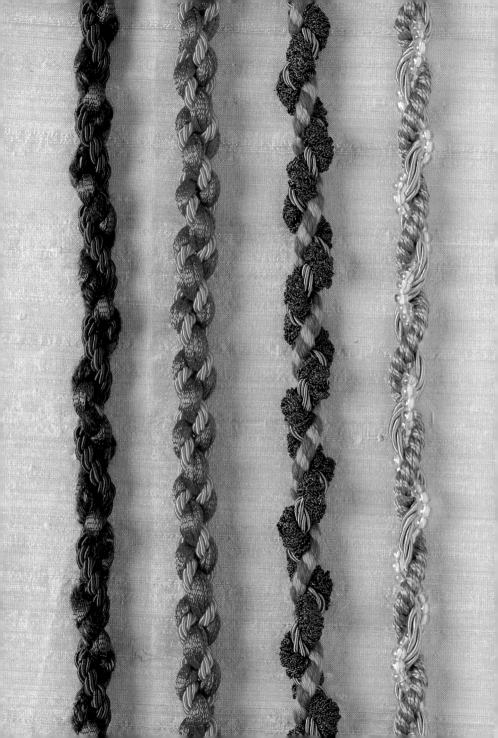

Three-ply

Twisting three elements together will make a three-ply cord. They can be S-twist or Z-twist depending on the direction of the helix.

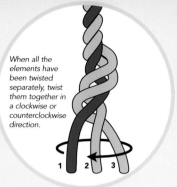

When all the elements have been twisted separately, twist them together in a clockwise or counterclockwise direction.

PLAIN
Easy rating ✔

Materials

Element 1 = 17 in (43 cm) = 12 strands of gray No 5 pearl cotton

Element 2 = 17 in (43 cm) = 12 strands of gray No 5 pearl cotton

Element 3 = 17 in (43 cm) = 12 strands of gray No 5 pearl cotton

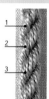

Method

Follow the instructions for Three-ply Cord (see page 28).

TWO COLORS
Easy rating ✔

Materials

Element 1 = 19 in (48 cm) 4 strands of purple Chunky wool

Element 2 = 19 in (48 cm) 4 strands of gray Chunky wool

Element 3 = 19 in (48 cm) 4 strands of gray Chunky wool

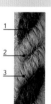

Method

Follow the instructions for Three-ply Cord (see page 28).

THREE COLORS
Easy rating ✔

Materials

Element 1 = 18 in (46 cm) = 4 strands of blue Double Top cotton

Element 2 = 18 in (46 cm) = 4 strands of mauve Double Top cotton

Element 3 = 18 in (46 cm) = 4 strands of purple Double Top cotton

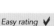

Method

Follow the instructions for Three-ply Cord (see page 28) but reverse the direction of the twist.

PLAIN AND BLENDED
Easy rating ✔

Materials

Element 1 = 17 in (43 cm) = 8 strands of mauve Double Top cotton

Element 2 = 17 in (43 cm) = 8 strands of mauve Double Top cotton

Element 3 = 17 in (43 cm) = 4 strands of blue and 4 strands of turquoise Double Top cotton

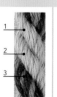

Method

Follow the instructions for Three-ply Cord (see page 28).

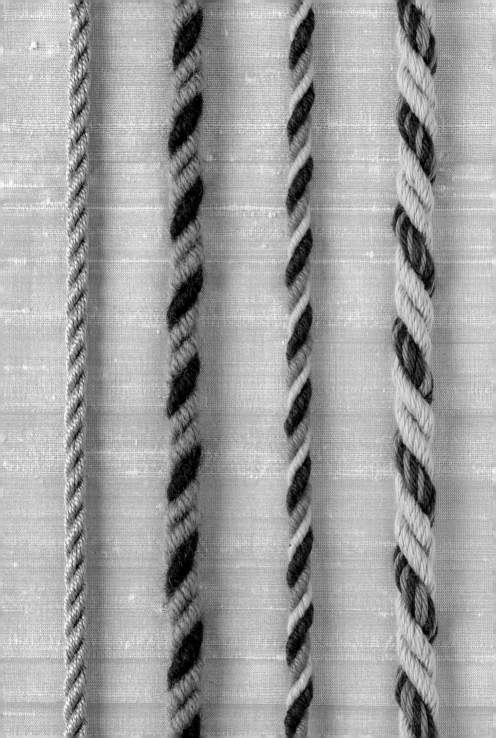

THREE THICKNESSES

Easy rating ✔

Materials

Element 1 = 16 in (41 cm) = 4 strands of dark gray No 5 pearl cotton

Element 2 = 16 in (41 cm) = 12 strands of gray No 5 pearl cotton

Element 3 = 16 in (41 cm) = 36 strands of light gray No 5 pearl cotton

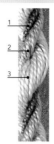

Method

Follow the instructions for Three-ply Cord (see page 28).

THREE TEXTURES

Easy rating ✔

Materials

Element 1 = 15 in (38 cm) = 2 strands of purple gimp

Element 2 = 15 in (38 cm) = 1 strand of purple lacing cord

Element 3 = 15 in (38 cm) = 16 strands of lilac Calmer cotton

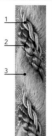

Method

Follow the instructions for Three-ply Cord (see page 28) but reverse the direction of the twist.

TWO TEXTURES

Easy rating ✔

Materials

Element 1 = 18 in (46 cm) = 4 strands of purple gimp

Element 2 = 18 in (46 cm) = 4 strands of mauve gimp

Element 3 = 18 in (46 cm) = 4 strands of gray wool

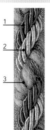

Method

Follow the instructions for Three-ply Cord (see page 28).

BEADS, WOOL, AND RIBBON

Easy rating ✔

Materials

Element 1 = 17 in (43 cm) = 6 strands of gray kid classic wool

Element 2 = 17 in (43 cm) = 6 strands of gray knitting ribbon

Element 3 = 17 in (43 cm) = 1 string of size 8° mauve rocaille beads

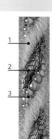

Method

Follow the instructions for Three-ply Cord (see page 28).

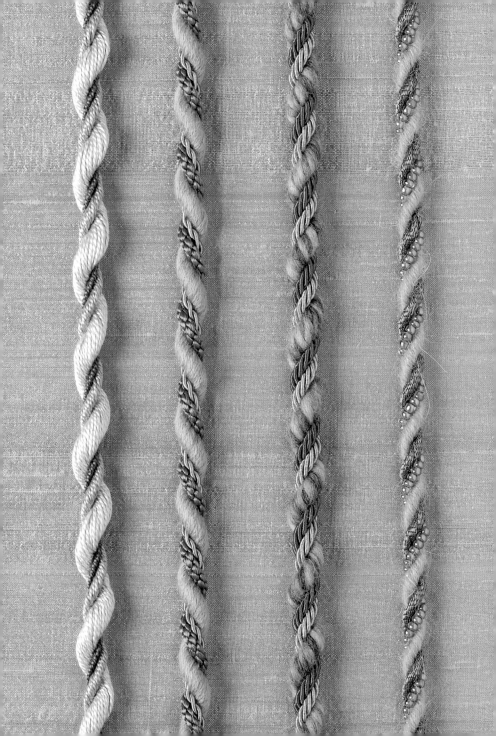

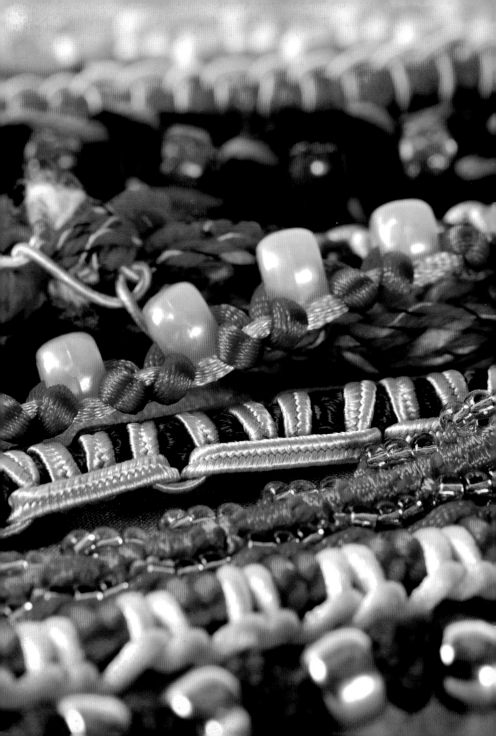

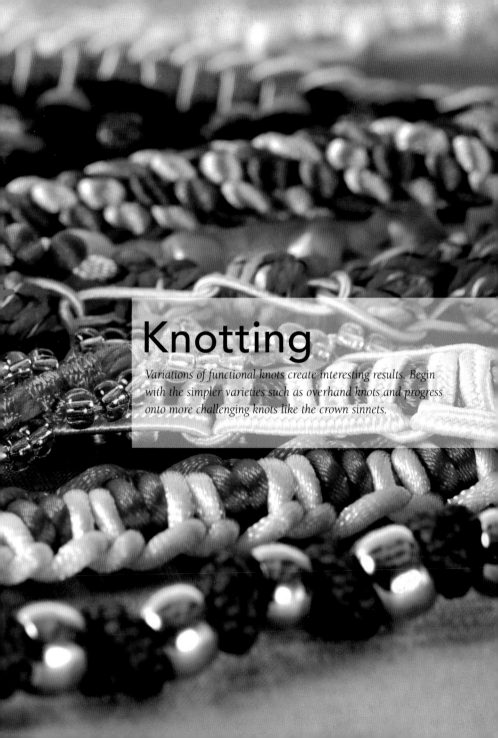

Knotting

Variations of functional knots create interesting results. Begin with the simpler varieties such as overhand knots and progress onto more challenging knots like the crown sinnets.

Overhand Knots

An Overhand Knot is one of the most basic knots. In fact it is sometimes called a simple knot. Here are three ways of working with overhand knots: in a single element, connecting the knots in a single element, and knots made over a core element.

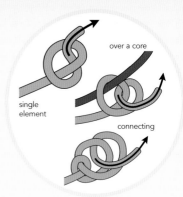

single element

over a core

connecting

PLAIN

Easy rating ✔

Materials
Element 1 = 28 in (71 cm) = 1 strand of ⅛-in (3-mm) diameter ocher lacing cord

Method
Make a series of Overhand Knots (see page 32) along the cord, leaving a small space between each.

PLAIN WITH BEADS

Easy rating ✔✔

Materials
Element 1 = 42 in (107 cm) = 1 strand of ⅛-in (3-mm) diameter terra-cotta lacing cord
25 gold pony beads

Method
Make an Overhand Knot (see page 32), then thread a pony bead onto the cord. Repeat this, pushing the knot close up to the bead every time.

CONNECTING, PLAIN

Easy rating ✔

Materials
Element 1 = 95 in (241 cm) = 1 strand of ⅟₁₆ in (2-mm) diameter gray rattail

Method
Make a series of Connecting Overhand Knots (see page 32).

OVER A CORE, TWO TEXTURES

Easy rating ✔

Materials
Element 1 = 12 in (30 cm) = 1 strand of ⅛-in (3-mm) diameter, terra-cotta lacing cord

Element 2 = 32 in (81 cm) = 8 strands of gray No 5 pearl cotton

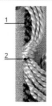

Method
Make a series of Overhand Knots Over a Core (see page 33). Leave a small space of about 1½ in (4 cm) between each knot. Gently pull Element 1, gathering up Element 2 to form soft loops.

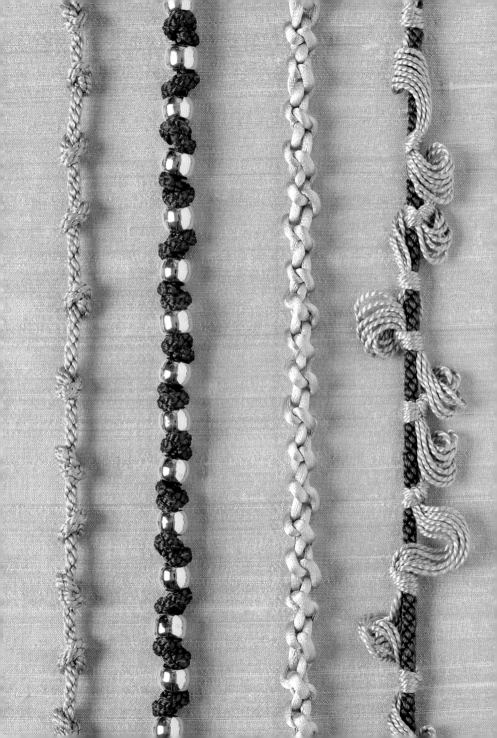

Half Hitches

Half hitches are made with two elements, one working over the other. They can be made in several ways and different effects can be created by working various combinations.

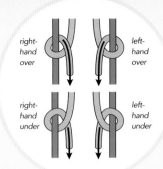

right-hand over

left-hand over

right-hand under

left-hand under

IDENTICAL, PLAIN

Easy rating ✔

Materials
Element 1 = 12 in (30 cm) = 1 strand of pink rattail. Element 1 is not visible

Element 2 = 92 in (234 cm) = 1 strand of pink rattail

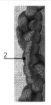

2

Method
The sample is made from a series of identical hitches. When the knots are pulled tight, the result will automatically form a spiral structure. Follow the instructions for a Series of Identical Half Hitches (see page 35).

IDENTICAL, TWO COLORS

Easy rating ✔✔

Materials
Element 1 = 12 in (30 cm) = 1 strand of burgundy Crepe cord

Element 2 = 81 in (206 cm) = 1 strand of pink Russia braid

1

2

Method
The sample is made from a series of identical hitches. Follow the instructions for a Series of Identical Half Hitches (see page 35) but do not tighten the knots. Keep the knots on the right-hand side and allow Element 1 to show through the structure.

OPPOSITE, PLAIN

Easy rating ✔

Materials
Element 1 = 12 in (30 cm) = 1 strand of pink rattail. Element 1 is not visible

Element 2 = 95 in (241 cm) = 1 strand of pink rattail

2

Method
This sample is made from opposite hitches. Follow the instructions for a Series of Opposite Half Hitches (see page 35).

OPPOSITE, TWO-COLOR WITH BEADS

Easy rating ✔

Materials
Element 1 = 12 in (30 cm) = 1 strand of gold rattail

Element 2 = 53 in (135 cm) = 1 strand of pink rattail threaded with 26 pink pony beads

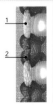

1

2

Method
This sample is made from opposite hitches. Follow the instructions for a Series of Opposite Half Hitches (see page 35). Push one bead up against the work after every pair of hitches.

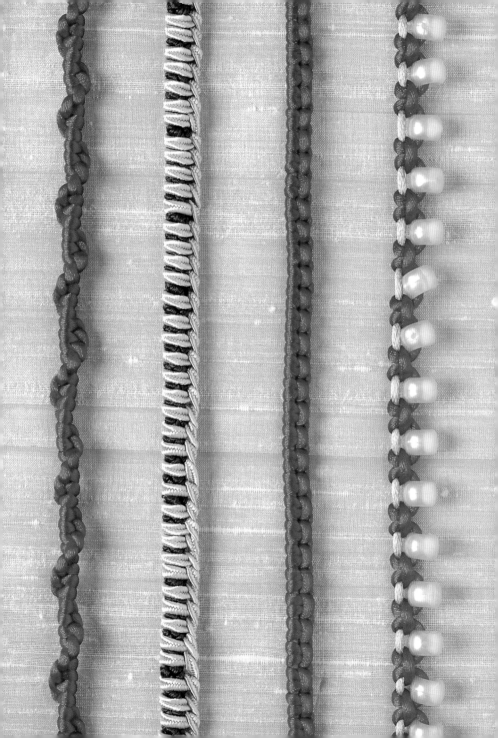

LEFT- AND RIGHT-HAND, PLAIN

Materials

Element 1 = 31 in (79 cm) = 1 strand of cream gimp

Element 2 = 31 in (79 cm) = 1 strand of cream gimp

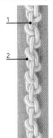

Method

This sample uses two elements but both the left- and the right-hand elements take it in turn to make the hitches, which creates a zigzag effect. Make a Series of Left- and Right-hand Half Hitches (see page 36). Do not pull the knots too tight.

LEFT- AND RIGHT-HAND, TWO COLORS

Materials

Element 1 = 38 in (97 cm) = 1 strand of ocher rattail

Element 2 = 38 in (97 cm) = 1 strand of pink rattail

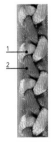

Method

This sample uses two elements but both the left- and the right-hand elements take it in turn to make the hitches, which creates a zigzag effect. Make a Series of Left- and Right-hand Half Hitches (see page 36). Do not pull the knots too tight.

LEFT- AND RIGHT-HAND, TWO TEXTURES

Materials

Element 1 = 29 in (74 cm) = 1 strand of ocher rattail

Element 2 = 33 in (84 cm) = 8 strands of pink Balmoral bouclé

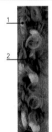

Method

This sample uses two elements but both the left- and the right-hand elements take it in turn to make the hitches, which creates a zigzag effect. Make a Series of Left- and Right-hand Half Hitches (see page 36). Do not pull the knots too tight.

LEFT- AND RIGHT-HAND, TWO TEXTURES

Materials

Element 1 = 32 in (81 cm) = 1 ocher, scallop-edged ribbon

Element 2 = 32 in (81 cm) = 1 strand of pink Chunky wool

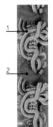

Method

This sample uses two elements but both the left- and the right-hand elements take it in turn to make the hitches, which creates a zigzag effect. Make a Series of Left- and Right-hand Half Hitches (see page 36). Do not pull the knots too tight. Try to keep the ribbon flat and evenly spaced. In this sample, three scallops were used for each hitch.

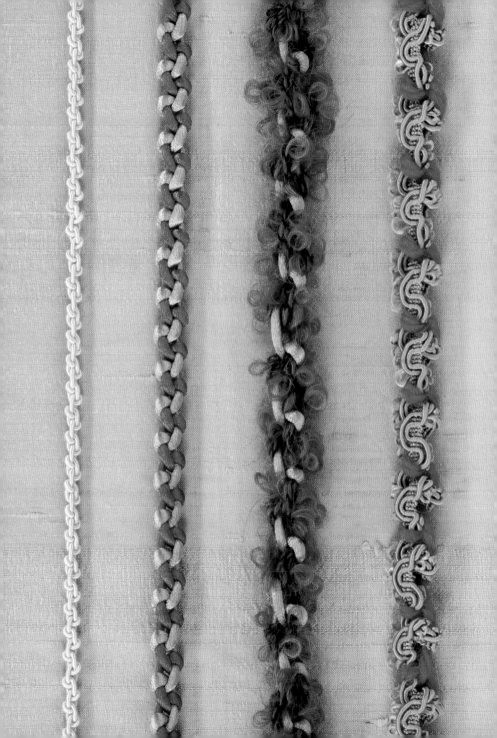

LEFT- AND RIGHT-HAND, OVER A CORE, PLAIN

Easy rating ✔

Materials

Element 1 = 82 in (208 cm) = 1 strand of ocher gimp

Element 2 = 12 in (30 cm) = 1 strand of ocher lacing cord. Element 2 is not visible

Element 3 = 82 in (208 cm) = 1 strand of ocher gimp

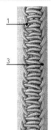

Method

This sample uses left- and right-hand hitches worked over a core element. Make a Series of Left- and Right-hand Half Hitches Over a Core (see page 37).

LEFT- AND RIGHT-HAND, OVER A CORE, TWO COLORS

Easy rating ✔

Materials

Element 1 = 77 in (196 cm) = 1 strand of pale pink Double Top cotton

Element 2 = 12 in (30 cm) = 4 strands of pink Double Top cotton. Element 2 is not visible

Element 3 = 77 in (196 cm) = 1 strand of pink Double Top cotton

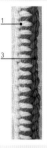

Method

This sample uses left- and right-hand hitches worked over a core element. Make a Series of Left- and Right-hand Half Hitches Over a Core (see page 37).

LEFT- AND RIGHT-HAND, OVER A CORE, TWO TEXTURES

Easy rating ✔

Materials

Element 1 = 52 in (132 cm) = 1 strand of pale pink gimp

Element 2 = 12 in (30 cm) = 4 strands of pink Double Top cotton. Element 2 is not visible

Element 3 = 65 in (165 cm) = 4 strands of pink knitting ribbon

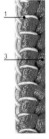

Method

This sample uses left- and right-hand hitches worked over a core element. Make a Series of Left- and Right-hand Half Hitches Over a Core (see page 37).

LEFT- AND RIGHT-HAND, OVER A CORE, TWO TEXTURES

Easy rating ✔

Materials

Element 1 = 33 in (84 cm) = 8 strands of Fancy Slub yarn (Festival)

Element 2 = 12 in (30 cm) = 1 strand of yellow gimp

Element 3 = 33 in (84 cm) = 1 strand of yellow gimp

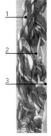

Method

This sample uses left- and right-hand hitches worked over a core element. Make a Series of Left- and Right-hand Half Hitches Over a Core (see page 37). Keep the knots loose so that the core can be seen.

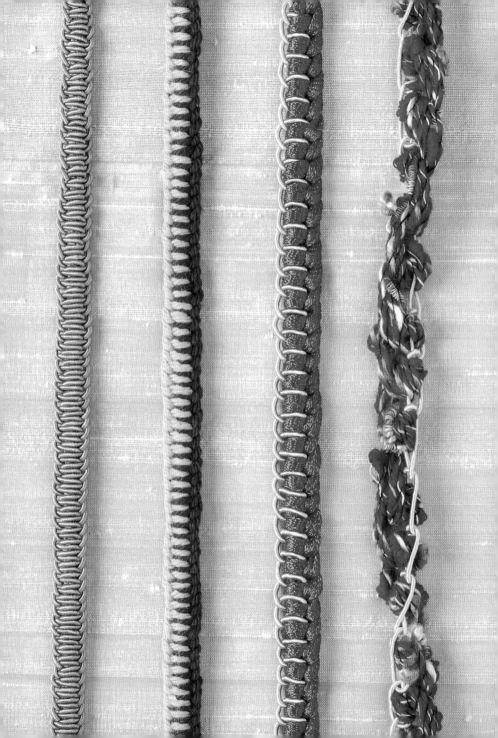

DOUBLE LEFT- AND RIGHT-HAND, OVER A CORE, PLAIN

Materials

Element 1 = 65 in (165 cm) = 1 strand of pale pink gimp

Element 2 = 12 in (30 cm) = 4 strands of pale pink Double Top cotton. Element 2 is not visible

Element 3 = 65 in (165 cm) = 1 strand of pale pink gimp

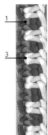

Method

This half hitch sample is similar to those on page 148, except each element works a pair of identical hitches over the core. Make a Series of Double Left- and Right-hand Half Hitches Over a Core (see page 38).

DOUBLE LEFT- AND RIGHT-HAND, OVER A CORE, TWO COLORS

Materials

Element 1 = 64 in (163 cm) = 1 strand of pink rattail

Element 2 = 12 in (30 cm) = 6 strands of pale pink Double Top cotton. Element 2 is not visible

Element 3 = 64 in (163 cm) = 1 strand of pale pink rattail

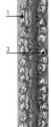

Method

This half hitch sample is similar to those on page 148, except each element works a pair of identical hitches over the core. Make a Series of Double Left- and Right-hand Half Hitches Over a Core (see page 38).

DOUBLE LEFT- AND RIGHT-HAND, OVER A CORE, BEADS AND RIBBON

Materials

Element 1 = 47 in (119 cm) = 1 strand of pink knitting ribbon, threaded with 27 gold size 6° beads

Element 2 = 12 in (30 cm) = 4 strands of pink Double Top cotton. Element 2 is not visible

Element 3 = 47 in (119 cm) = 1 strand of pink knitting ribbon, threaded with 27 gold size 6° beads

Method

The beads are added during a Series of Double Left- and Right-hand Half Hitches Over a Core (see page 38). Push three beads up to the top of Element 3, then make two Right-hand Over Half Hitches over Element 2, making sure that the beads remain above the hitches. Push three beads up to the top of Element 1 and make two Left-hand Over Half Hitches over Element 2, making sure that the beads remain above the hitches.

DOUBLE LEFT- AND RIGHT-HAND, OVER A CORE, BEADS AND GIMP

Materials

Element 1 = 32 in (81 cm) = 1 strand pink gimp

Element 2 = 12 in (30 cm) = 4 strands of pale pink Double Top cotton, threaded with 8 gold lozenge beads

Element 3 = 32 in (81 cm) = 1 strand of pink gimp

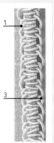

Method

The beads are added during a Series of Double Left- and Right-hand Half Hitches Over a Core (see page 38). A bead is pushed up the core after every 8 hitches (4 pairs).

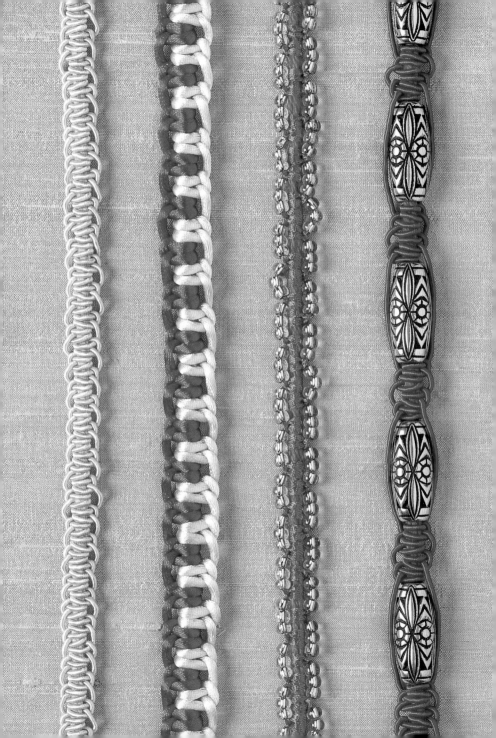

DOUBLE LEFT- AND RIGHT-HAND, OPPOSITE, OVER A CORE, PLAIN

Easy rating ✔

Materials

Element 1 = 45 in (114 cm) = 1 strand of pale pink rattail

Element 2 = 12 in (30 cm) = 1 strand of pale pink rattail. Element 2 is not visible

Element 3 = 45 in (114 cm) = 1 strand of pale pink rattail

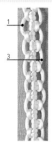

Method

Each left- and right-hand element works a pair of hitches over the core element. However, the pair of hitches work in opposite directions. Make a Series of Double Left- and Right-hand Opposite Half Hitches Over a Core (see page 39).

DOUBLE LEFT- AND RIGHT-HAND, OPPOSITE, OVER A CORE, TWO COLORS

Easy rating ✔

Materials

Element 1 = 54 in (137 cm) = 1 strand of pale pink Double Top cotton

Element 2 = 12 in (30 cm) = 1 strand of brown Double Top cotton. Element 2 is not visible

Element 3 = 54 in (137 cm) = 1 strand of brown Double Top cotton

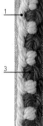

Method

Each left- and right-hand element works a pair of hitches over the core element. However, the pair of hitches work in opposite directions. Make a Series of Double Left- and Right-hand Opposite Half Hitches Over a Core (see page 39).

DOUBLE LEFT- AND RIGHT-HAND, OPPOSITE, OVER A CORE, CORE REVEALED

Easy rating ✔

Materials

Element 1 = 37 in (94 cm) = 1 strand of pink Russia braid

Element 2 = 12 in (30 cm) = 1 strand of brown Crepe cord

Element 3 = 37 in (94 cm) = 1 strand of pink Russia braid

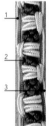

Method

Each left- and right-hand element works a pair of hitches over the core element. However, the pair of hitches work in opposite directions. Make a Series of Double Left- and Right-hand Opposite Half Hitches Over a Core (see page 39). Spread the hitches out so that the core Element 2 shows.

DOUBLE LEFT- AND RIGHT-HAND, OPPOSITE, OVER A CORE, THREE TEXTURES

Easy rating ✔

Materials

Element 1 = 39 in (99 cm) = 1 strand of pale pink gimp

Element 2 = 12 in (30 cm) = 1 strand of brown lacing cord. Element 2 is not visible

Element 3 = 49 in (124 cm) = 4 strands of pink Balmoral bouclé

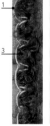

Method

Each left- and right-hand element works a pair of hitches over the core element. However, the pair of hitches work in opposite directions. Make a Series of Double Left- and Right-hand Opposite Half Hitches Over a Core (see page 39).

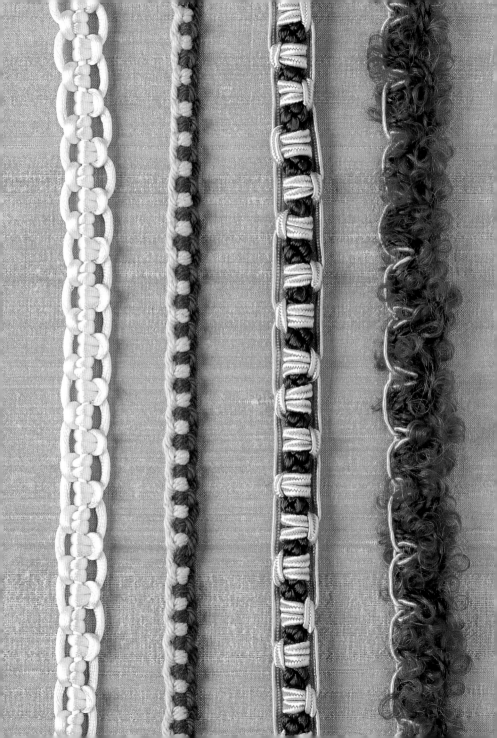

Half Knots

Half knots differ from hitches in that both of the two elements work equally. They can be made more solid by being worked over a core element. The technique falls under the category of Macramé, or Square Knotting. This beautiful spiral structure is made from a series of identical half knots over a core. It is known as a Barrister Bar, Twisted Bar, or Spiral Sennit. The knots twist as you work, so don't try to stop them.

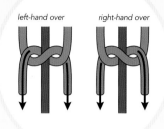

left-hand over   *right-hand over*

IDENTICAL, OVER A CORE, PLAIN

Easy rating ✔

Materials

Element 1 = 57 in (145 cm) = 1 strand of blue rattail

Element 2 = 12 in (30 cm) = 1 strand of blue rattail. Element 2 is not visible

Element 3 = 57 in (145 cm) = 1 strand of blue rattail

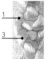

Method

Make a Series of Identical Half Knots over a Core (see page 40).

IDENTICAL, OVER A CORE, TWO COLORS

Easy rating ✔

Materials

Element 1 = 57 in (145 cm) = 1 strand of navy gimp

Element 2 = 12 in (30 cm) = 1 strand of navy gimp. Element 2 is not visible

Element 3 = 57 in (145 cm) = 1 strand of blue gimp

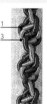

Method

Make a Series of Identical Half Knots Over a Core (see page 40).

IDENTICAL, OVER A CORE, THICK CORE

Easy rating ✔

Materials

Element 1 = 91 in (231 cm) = 1 strand of blue Double Top cotton

Element 2 = 12 in (30 cm) = 1 strand of navy crepe cord. Element 2 is not visible.

Element 3 = 91 in (231 cm) = 1 strand of turquoise Double Top cotton

Method

Make a Series of Identical Half Knots Over a Core (see page 40).

IDENTICAL, OVER A CORE, BEADS AND TEXTURE

Easy rating ✔✔

Materials

Element 1 = 46 in (117 cm) = 1 strand of blue lacing cord

Element 2 = 12 in (30 cm) = 26 strands of No 5 pearl cotton threaded with 21 pony beads

Element 3 = 56 in (142 cm) = 1 strand of turquoise Double Top cotton

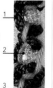

Method

The beads are added during a Series of Identical Half Knots Over a Core (see page 40). Push a bead up the core after every three hitches.

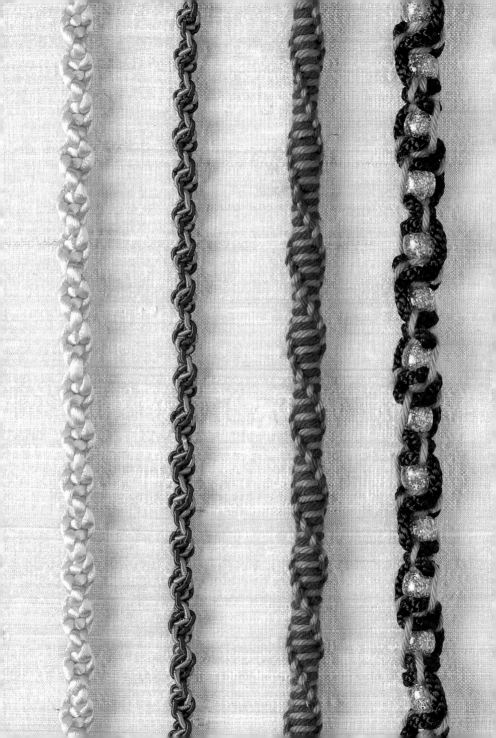

OPPOSITE, OVER A CORE, PLAIN

Easy rating ✔
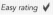

Materials
Element 1 = 57 in (145 cm) = 1 strand of turquoise gimp

Element 2 = 12 in (30 cm) = 1 strand of turquoise gimp

Element 3 = 57 in (145 cm) = 1 strand of turquoise gimp

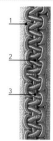

Method
Opposite half knots can be made over a core with the left-hand and right-hand elements taking it in turn to make the first loop. These are the equivalent of reef knots made around the core. The structure is known as a Solomon's Bar or Flat Sennit. Make a Series of Opposite Half Knots Over a Core (see page 42).

OPPOSITE, OVER A CORE, TWO COLORS

Easy rating ✔

Materials
Element 1 = 57 in (145 cm) = 1 strand of blue rattail

Element 2 = 12 in (30 cm) = 1 strand of ocher rattail

Element 3 = 57 in (145 cm) = 1 strand of ocher rattail

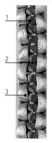

Method
Opposite half knots can be made over a core with the left-hand and right-hand elements taking it in turn to make the first loop. These are the equivalent of reef knots made around the core. The structure is known as a Solomon's Bar or Flat Sennit. Make a Series of Opposite Half Knots Over a Core (see page 42).

OPPOSITE, OVER A CORE, BEADS AND COTTON

Easy rating ✔✔

Materials
Element 1 = 53 in (135 cm) = 2 strands of turquoise No 8 pearl cotton threaded with 60 size 6° frosted rocailles

Element 2 = 12 in (30 cm) = 1 strand of navy lacing cord

Element 3 = 53 in (135 cm) = 2 strands of turquoise No 8 pearl cotton threaded with 60 size 6° frosted rocailles

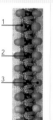

Method
Opposite half knots can be made over a core with the left-hand and right-hand elements taking it in turn to make the first loop. These are the equivalent of reef knots made around the core. The structure is known as a Solomon's Bar or Flat Sennit. The beads are added during a Series of Opposite Half Knots Over a Core (see page 42). Push a bead up from both Elements 1 and 3 before making each pair of opposite half knots.

OPPOSITE, OVER A CORE, THICK AND THIN

Easy rating ✔

Materials
Element 1 = 57 in (145 cm) = 1 strand of turquoise Double Top cotton

Element 2 = 12 in (30 cm) = 1 strand of ocher lacing cord

Element 3 = 47 in (119 cm) = 1 strand of navy lacing cord

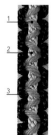

Method
Opposite half knots can be made over a core with the left-hand and right-hand elements taking it in turn to make the first loop. These are the equivalent of reef knots made around the core. The structure is known as a Solomon's Bar or Flat Sennit. Make a Series of Opposite Half Knots Over a Core (see page 42). Keep the navy lacing cord on the upper surface of the knotting.

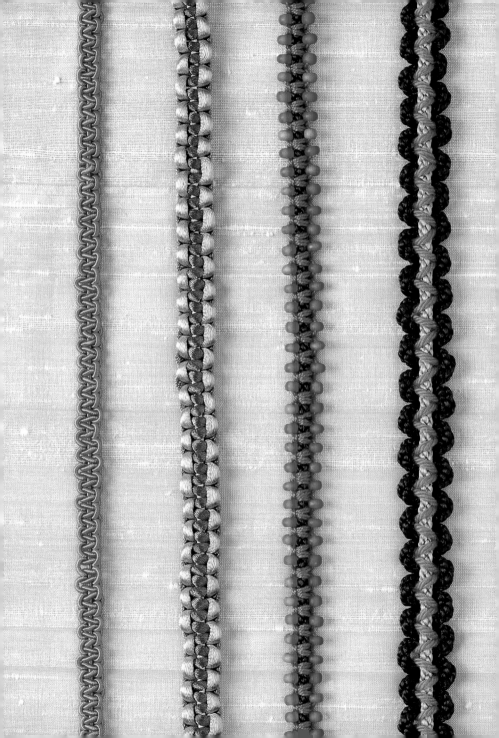

Crown Sinnets

These Crown Sinnets are made with four elements that are folded over each other, with the last element taken through the loop made by the first element. The technique is also known as Scoobee Doo when made with plastic tubing. These samples produce a round structure and are made by "crowning" in the same direction (counterclockwise). Various patterns can be produced by having the colored elements starting in different positions.

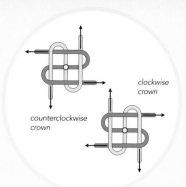

clockwise crown

counterclockwise crown

IDENTICAL, PLAIN

Easy rating ✔✔

Materials

Element 1 = 45 in (114 cm) = 1 strand of pink plastic tubing

Element 2 = 45 in (114 cm) = 1 strand of pink plastic tubing

Element 3 = 45 in (114 cm) = 1 strand of pink plastic tubing

Element 4 = 45 in (114 cm) = 1 strand of pink plastic tubing

Method

Make a Series of Identical Crowns (see page 44).

IDENTICAL, OVER A CORE, TWO COLORS, 1:3

Easy rating ✔✔

Materials

Element 1 = 53 in (135 cm) = 1 strand of gold rattail

Element 2 = 53 in (135 cm) = 1 strand of purple rattail

Element 3 = 53 in (135 cm) = 1 strand of purple rattail

Element 4 = 53 in (135 cm) = 1 strand of purple rattail

Method

Make a Series of Identical Crowns (see page 44).

IDENTICAL, TWO COLORS, 2:2 ADJACENT

Easy rating ✔✔

Materials

Element 1 = 45 in (114 cm) = 1 strand of purple plastic tubing

Element 2 = 45 in (114 cm) = 1 strand of purple plastic tubing

Element 3 = 45 in (114 cm) = 1 strand of yellow plastic tubing

Element 4 = 45 in (114 cm) = 1 strand of yellow plastic tubing

Method

Make a Series of Identical Crowns (see page 44).

IDENTICAL, TWO COLORS, 2:2 OPPOSITE

Easy rating ✔✔

Materials

Element 1 = 53 in (135 cm) = 1 strand of mauve rattail

Element 2 = 53 in (135 cm) = 1 strand of purple rattail

Element 3 = 53 in (135 cm) = 1 strand of mauve rattail

Element 4 = 53 in (135 cm) = 1 strand of purple rattail

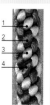

Method

Make a series of Identical Crowns (see page 44) working the elements in a counterclockwise direction.

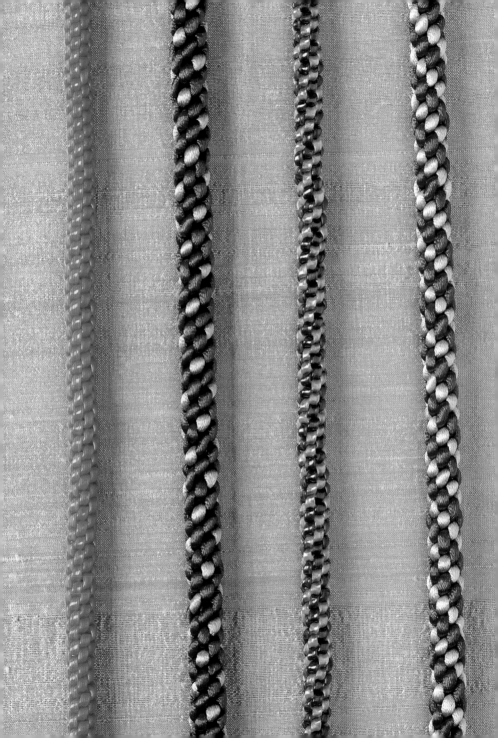

IDENTICAL, THREE COLORS 1:1:2 ADJACENT

Easy rating ✔✔

Materials

Element 1 = 53 in (135 cm) = 1 strand of mauve rattail

Element 2 = 53 in (135 cm) = 1 strand of mauve rattail

Element 3 = 53 in (135 cm) = 1 strand of blue rattail

Element 4 = 53 in (135 cm) = 1 strand of purple rattail

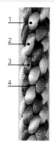

Method

Make a Series of Identical Crowns (see page 44).

IDENTICAL, THREE COLORS 1:1:2 OPPOSITE

Easy rating ✔✔

Materials

Element 1 = 53 in (135 cm) = 1 strand of brown rattail

Element 2 = 53 in (135 cm) = 1 strand of pink rattail

Element 3 = 53 in (135 cm) = 1 strand of brown rattail

Element 4 = 53 in (135 cm) = 1 strand of gold rattail

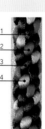

Method

Make a Series of Identical Crowns (see page 44).

IDENTICAL, FOUR COLORS

Easy rating ✔✔

Materials

Element 1 = 53 in (135 cm) = 1 strand of pink rattail

Element 2 = 53 in (135 cm) = 1 strand of purple rattail

Element 3 = 53 in (135 cm) = 1 strand of gold rattail

Element 4 = 53 in (135 cm) = 1 strand of blue rattail

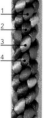

Method

Make a Series of Identical Crowns (see page 44).

IDENTICAL, BEADS AND RATTAIL

Easy rating ✔✔

Materials

Element 1 = 51 in (130 cm) = 1 strand of gold rattail

Element 2 = 31 in (79 cm) = 1 string of size 8° beads

Element 3 = 51 in (130 cm) = 1 strand of gold rattail

Element 4 = 31 in (79 cm) = 1 string of size 8° beads

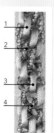

Method

Make a Series of Identical Crowns (see page 44). Do not pull the elements too tightly.

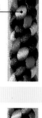

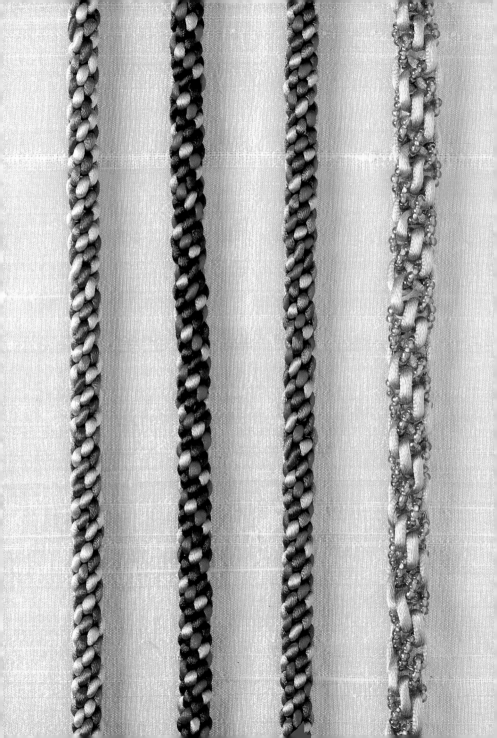

OPPOSITE, PLAIN

Materials

Element 1 = 47 in (119 cm) = 1 strand of purple plastic tubing

Element 2 = 47 in (119 cm) = 1 strand of purple plastic tubing

Element 3 = 47 in (119 cm) = 1 strand of purple plastic tubing

Element 4 = 47 in (119 cm) = 1 strand of purple plastic tubing

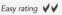
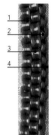

Method

A square structure can be created by working crowns alternately clockwise and counterclockwise. This is sometimes called "reverse crowning." Make a Series of Opposite Crowns (see page 46).

OPPOSITE, TWO COLORS 2:2 OPPOSITE

Materials

Element 1 = 40 in (102 cm) = 1 strand of purple Chunky wool

Element 2 = 40 in (102 cm) = 1 strand of mauve Chunky wool

Element 3 = 40 in (102 cm) = 1 strand of purple Chunky wool

Element 4 = 40 in (102 cm) = 1 strand of mauve Chunky wool

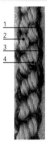

Method

A square structure can be created by working crowns alternately clockwise and counterclockwise. This is sometimes called "reverse crowning." Make a Series of Opposite Crowns (see page 46). Do not pull too hard, as the wool is very stretchy.

OPPOSITE, TWO COLORS 2:2 ADJACENT

Materials

Element 1 = 47 in (119 cm) = 1 strand of purple rattail

Element 2 = 47 in (119 cm) = 1 strand of purple rattail

Element 3 = 47 in (119 cm) = 1 strand of gold rattail

Element 4 = 47 in (119 cm) = 1 strand of gold rattail

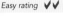
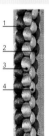

Method

A square structure can be created by working crowns alternately clockwise and counterclockwise. This is sometimes called "reverse crowning." Make a Series of Opposite Crowns (see page 46).

OPPOSITE, THREE COLORS 1:1:2 OPPOSITE

Materials

Element 1 = 47 in (119 cm) = 1 strand of ocher rattail

Element 2 = 47 in (119 cm) = 1 strand of brown rattail

Element 3 = 47 in (119 cm) = 1 strand of ocher rattail

Element 4 = 47 in (119 cm) = 1 strand of pink rattail

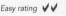
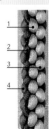

Method

A square structure can be created by working crowns alternately clockwise and counterclockwise. This is sometimes called "reverse crowning." Make a Series of Opposite Crowns (see page 46).

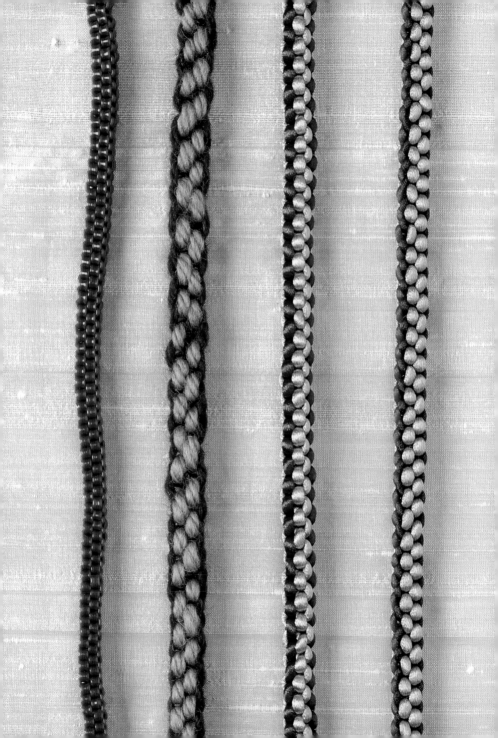

OPPOSITE, THREE COLORS 1:1:2 ADJACENT

Easy rating ✔✔

Materials

Element 1 = 53 in (135 cm) = 1 strand of ocher rattail

Element 2 = 53 in (135 cm) = 1 strand of ocher rattail

Element 3 = 53 in (135 cm) = 1 strand of brown rattail

Element 4 = 53 in (135 cm) = 1 strand of burgundy rattail

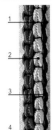

Method

A square structure can be created by working crowns alternately clockwise and counterclockwise. This is sometimes called "reverse crowning." Make a Series of Opposite Crowns (see page 46).

OPPOSITE, FOUR COLORS

Easy rating ✔✔

Materials

Element 1 = 47 in (119 cm) = 1 strand of blue rattail

Element 2 = 47 in (119 cm) = 1 strand of purple rattail

Element 3 = 47 in (119 cm) =1 strand of pink rattail

Element 4 = 47 in (119 cm) = 1 strand of ocher rattail

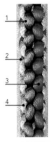

Method

A square structure can be created by working crowns alternately clockwise and counterclockwise. This is sometimes called "reverse crowning." Make a Series of Opposite Crowns (see page 46).

OPPOSITE, TWO TEXTURES

Easy rating ✔✔

Materials

Element 1 = 43 in (109 cm) = 1 strand of ocher lacing cord

Element 2 = 40 in (102 cm) = 1 strand of ocher lacing cord

Element 3 = 40 in (102 cm) = 1 strand of purple rattail

Element 4 = 40 in (102 cm) = 1 strand of purple rattail

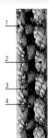

Method

A square structure can be created by working crowns alternately clockwise and counterclockwise. This is sometimes called "reverse crowning." Make a Series of Opposite Crowns (see page 46).

OPPOSITE, RIBBON

Easy rating ✔✔✔

Materials

Element 1 = 108 in (274 cm) = 1 strand of purple ribbon

Element 2 = 108 in (274 cm) = 1 strand of purple ribbon

Element 3 = 108 in (274 cm) = 1 strand of purple ribbon

Element 4 = 108 in (274 cm) = 1 strand of purple ribbon

Method

A square structure can be created by working crowns alternately clockwise and counterclockwise. This is sometimes called "reverse crowning." Make a Series of Opposite Crowns (see page 46). Fold the ribbon so that it remains flat.

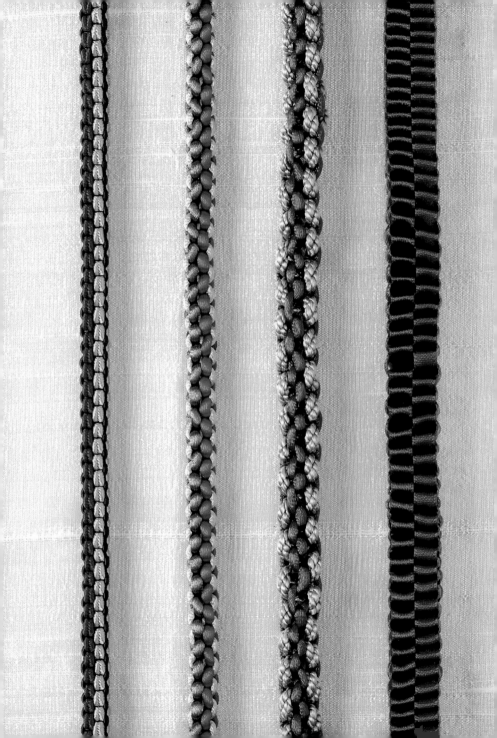

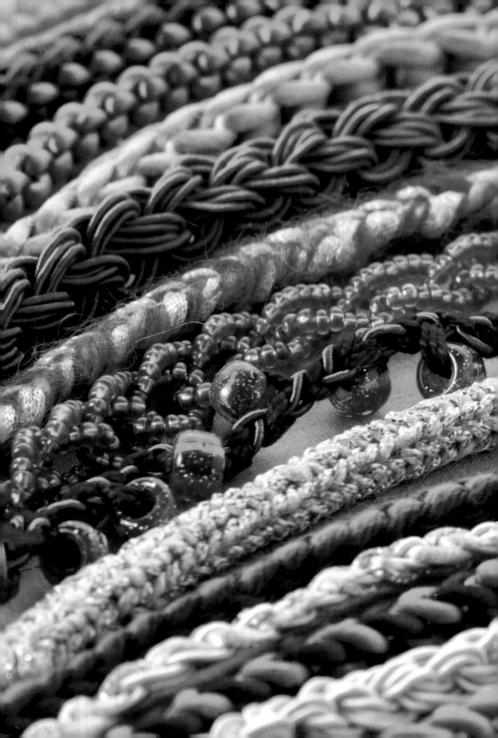

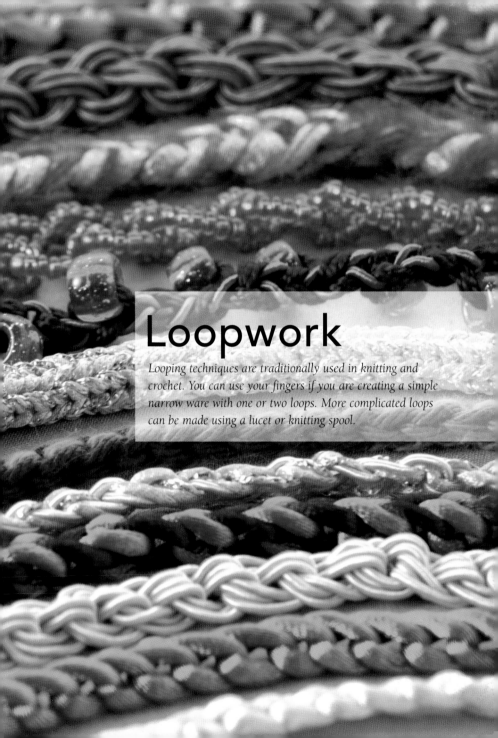

Loopwork

Looping techniques are traditionally used in knitting and crochet. You can use your fingers if you are creating a simple narrow ware with one or two loops. More complicated loops can be made using a lucet or knitting spool.

One Element, One Loop

There are many ways of interlooping with a single element. A one-loop version is the most basic. This simple narrow ware is easy to make and is known by many names such as Chain Sinnet, Monkey Braid, Trumpet Cord, and Crochet Stitch.

The element comes from below each time and makes a new loop.

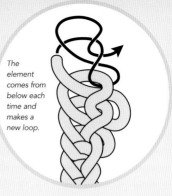

PLAIN

Easy rating ✔

Materials
Element 1 = 69 in (175 cm) = 1 strand of peach rattail

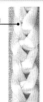

Method
Follow the instructions for One Element, One Loop (see page 49).

WITH BEADS

Easy rating ✔✔

Materials
Element 1 = 52 in (132 cm) = 1 string of size 8° peach rocaille beads

Method
Follow the instructions for One Element, One Loop (see page 49) but do not pull the stitches too tight.

TEXTURE

Easy rating ✔✔

Materials
Element 1 = 61 in (155 cm) = 3 strands of cream gimp

Method
Follow the instructions for One Element, One Loop (see page 49). Take care to keep all strands together as one element.

TEXTURE

Easy rating ✔✔

Materials
Element 1 = 59 in (150 cm) = 1 strand of peach knitting ribbon, 1 strand of yellow Glitter, and 1 strand of cream gimp

Method
Follow the instructions for One Element, One Loop (see page 49). Take care to keep all strands together as one element.

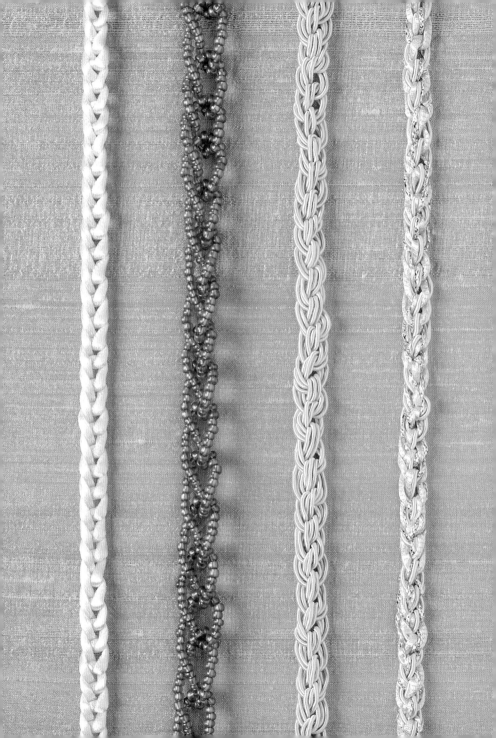

One Element, Two Loops

There are more possibilities for making two-loop versions with just one element. Two variations are shown on the opposite page. The first and third samples are usually made on a lucet and are known as Square Loop Sinnets. The second and fourth samples interloop hitches to produce a flatter structure.

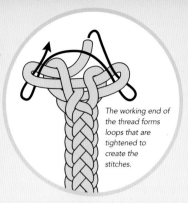

The working end of the thread forms loops that are tightened to create the stitches.

PLAIN

Easy rating ✔

Materials
Element 1 = 121 in (307 cm) = 1 strand of peach rattail

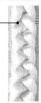

Method
Follow the instructions for One Element, Two Loops (see page 50).

WITH HITCHES, PLAIN

Easy rating ✔

Materials
Element 1 = 127 in (323 cm) = 1 strand of pink rattail

Method
Follow the instructions for One Element, Two Loops with Hitches (see page 54).

TEXTURE

Easy rating ✔

Materials
Element 1 = 118 in (300 cm) = 1 strand of Biggy Print wool

Method
Follow the instructions for One Element, Two Loops (see page 50).

WITH HITCHES, TEXTURE

Easy rating ✔✔

Materials
Element 1 = 137 in (348 cm) = 2 strands of pink knitting ribbon and 4 strands of Kidsilk Haze

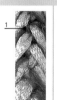

Method
Follow the instructions for One Element, Two Loops with Hitches (see page 54). Take care to keep all the strands acting as one element.

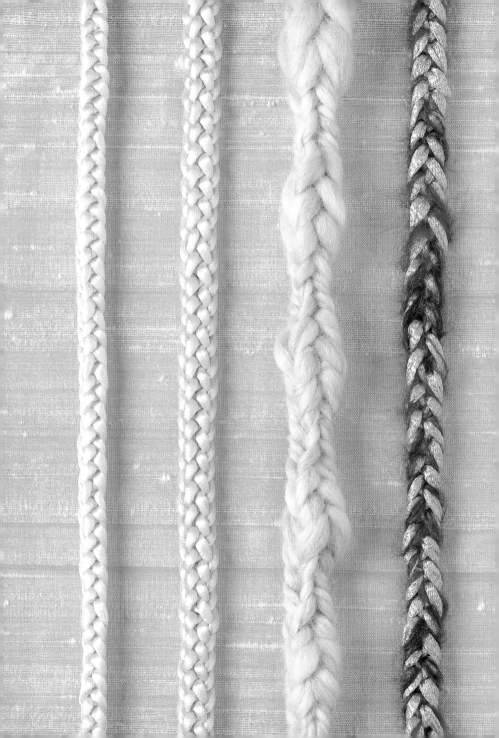

One Element, Four Loops

The four-loop round version is a popular technique, usually made on a Knitting Nancy. The work has many names, such as French Knitting, Corking, Rat's Tails, and Peg Knitting. The flat version is also worked on the Knitting Nancy. It is just like a very narrow section of plain knitting.

In both the round and the flat versions the threads go on a journey around the pegs (see pages 56–59).

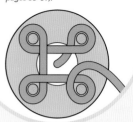

ROUND, PLAIN

Easy rating ✔

Materials
Element 1 = 258 in (655 cm) = 1 strand of peach Double Top cotton

Method
Follow the instructions for One Element, Four Loops, Round (see page 56).

ROUND, TEXTURE

Easy rating ✔✔

Materials
Element 1 = 307 in (780 cm) = 1 strand of peach knitting ribbon and 1 strand of Glitter

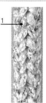

Method
Follow the instructions for One Element, Four Loops, Round (see page 56). Take care to pick up both strands together when making the loops.

FLAT, PLAIN

Easy rating ✔

Materials
Element 1 = 237 in (602 cm) = 1 strand of peach Double Top cotton

Method
Follow the instructions for One Element, Four Loops, Flat (see page 58).

FLAT, TEXTURE

Easy rating ✔✔

Materials
Element 1 = 229 in (582 cm) = 1 strand of Tinsel

Method
Follow the instructions for One Element, Four Loops, Flat (see page 58).

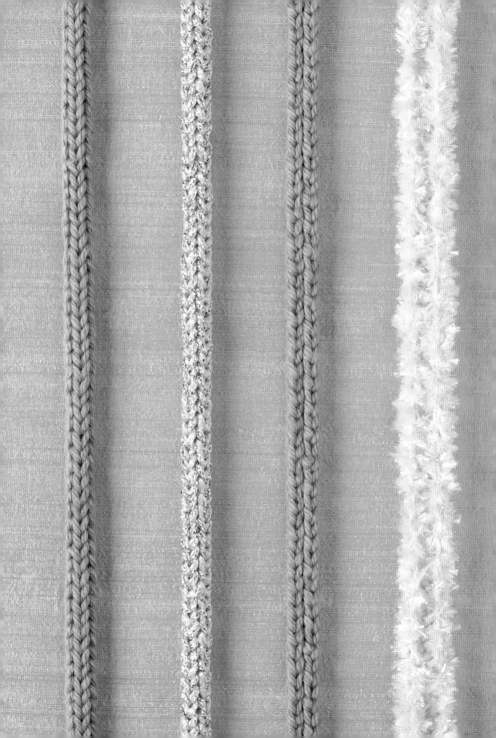

Two Elements, One Loop

Two elements interlooped together give the possibility of pattern. These samples use a single loop, drawing up each element alternately. The structure has many names including Double Loop Chain, Serbian Cord, Crochet Cord, and Idiot's Delight.

The two elements are worked together by taking them alternately through a single loop.

PLAIN
Easy rating ✔

Materials
Element 1 = 54 in (137 cm) = 1 strand of green rattail

Element 2 = 54 in (137 cm) = 1 strand of green rattail

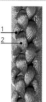

Method
Follow the instructions for Two Elements, One Loop (see page 60).

TWO COLORS
Easy rating ✔

Materials
Element 1 = 53 in (135 cm) = 1 strand of burgandy rattail

Element 2 = 53 in (135 cm) = 1 strand of green rattail

Method
Follow the instructions for Two Elements, One Loop (see page 60).

RIBBON
Easy rating ✔✔

Materials
Element 1 = 53 in (135 cm) = 1 strand of burgundy ribbon

Element 2 = 53 in (135 cm) = 1 strand of green ribbon

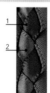

Method
Follow the instructions for Two Elements, One Loop (see page 60). Fold the ribbon to keep it flat. You might find it easier to make each new loop by pushing a fold of the ribbon up through the previous loop (rather than pulling it up).

GIMP
Easy rating ✔

Materials
Element 1 = 43 in (109 cm) = 4 strands of green gimp

Element 2 = 43 in (109 cm) = 4 strands of green gimp

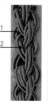

Method
Follow the instructions for Two Elements, One Loop (see page 60).

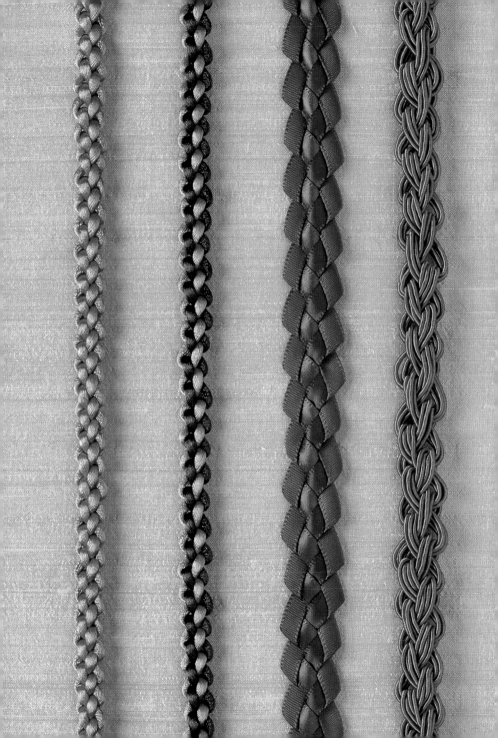

Two Elements, One Loop, Triangular

These two-element, one-loop samples also draw up alternate loops from two elements. However, the finished product has three ridges, giving a more triangular-looking cross section.

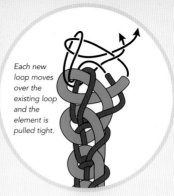

Each new loop moves over the existing loop and the element is pulled tight.

TRIANGULAR, PLAIN

Easy rating ✔

Materials

Element 1 = 43 in (109 cm) = 1 strand of green rattail

Element 2 = 43 in (109 cm) = 1 strand of green rattail

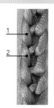

Method
Follow the instructions for Two Elements, One Loop, Triangular (see page 62).

TRIANGULAR, TWO COLORS

Easy rating ✔

Materials

Element 1 = 43 in (109 cm) = 1 strand of green rattail

Element 2 = 43 in (109 cm) = 1 strand of burgundy rattail

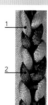

Method
Follow the instructions for Two Elements, One Loop, Triangular (see page 62).

TRIANGULAR, TWO TEXTURES

Easy rating ✔

Materials

Element 1 = 34 in (86 cm) = 1 strand of green ruched knitting ribbon

Element 2 = 46 in (117 cm) = 1 strand of burgundy Russia braid

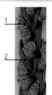

Method
Follow the instructions for Two Elements, One Loop, Triangular (see page 62). Keep tension loose and flatten the finished result.

TRIANGULAR, TWO COLORS WITH BEADS

Easy rating ✔✔

Materials

Element 1 = 43 in (109 cm) = 1 strand of green gimp

Element 2 = 47 in (119 cm) = 4 strands of burgundy No 5 pearl cotton, threaded with 20 green pony beads

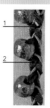

Method
Follow the instructions for Two Elements, One Loop, Triangular (see page 62). A bead is added every alternate move with Element 2. Before the loop is made with Element 2, push the bead close up against the work. Make sure it stays close to the work and does not become part of the loop.

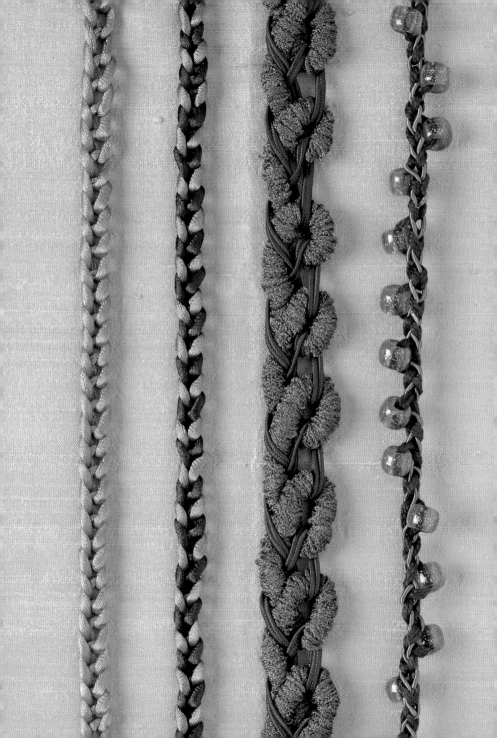

Two Elements, Two Loops

Here two loops are used, with each element working through its own loop. In fact, they are two Chain Sinnets (One Element, One Loop) connecting together with a cross at the center.

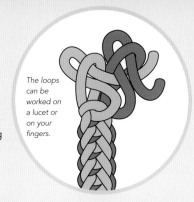

The loops can be worked on a lucet or on your fingers.

PLAIN

Easy rating ✔

Materials
Element 1 = 58 in (147 cm) = 1 strand of ocher rattail

Element 2 = 58 in (147 cm) = 1 strand of ocher rattail

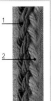

Method
Follow the instructions for Two Elements, Two Loops (see page 64).

TWO COLORS

Easy rating ✔

Materials
Element 1 = 59 in (150 cm) = 1 strand of green Double Top cotton

Element 2 = 59 in (150 cm) = 1 strand of light green Double Top cotton

Method
Follow the instructions for Two Elements, Two Loops (see page 64).

RUSSIA BRAID

Easy rating ✔✔

Materials
Element 1 = 65 in (165 cm) = 1 strand of ocher Russia braid

Element 2 = 65 in (165 cm) = 1 strand of green Russia braid

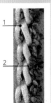

Method
Follow the instructions for Two Elements, Two Loops (see page 64). Keep the braid flat around the fingers or pegs.

TWO TEXTURES

Easy rating ✔

Materials
Element 1 = 59 in (150 cm) = 1 strand of ocher rattail

Element 2 = 49 in (124 cm) = 1 strand of green Fancy wool

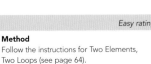

Method
Follow the instructions for Two Elements, Two Loops (see page 64).

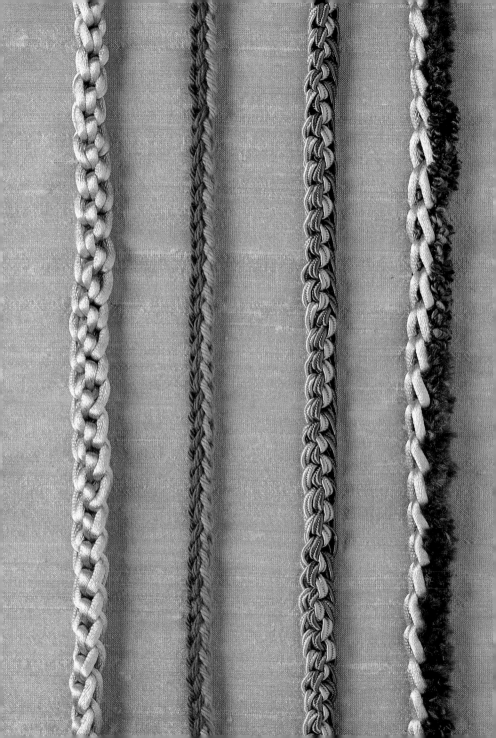

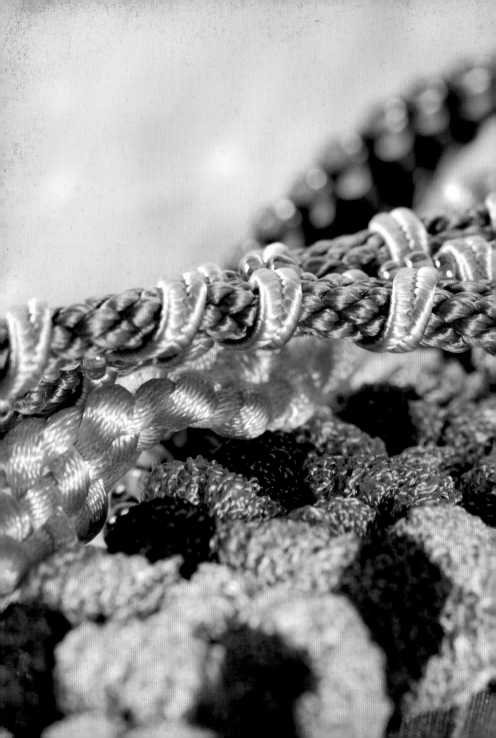

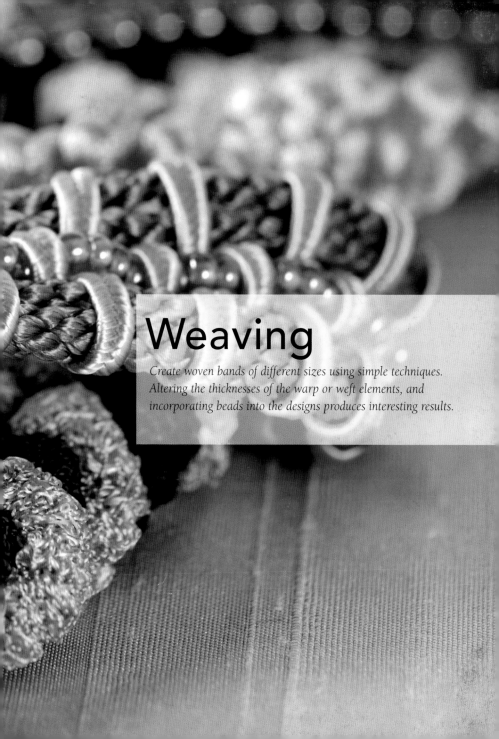

Weaving

Create woven bands of different sizes using simple techniques. Altering the thicknesses of the warp or weft elements, and incorporating beads into the designs produces interesting results.

Two Warps

The narrowest form of weaving is made with a weft interlacing over and under just two warps. Its common form is weft-faced, with the warps completely hidden from view (see Two Warps, Weft-faced, page 186). It has been called many names including Overcasting, Wrapped Braid, Needlewoven Braid, and Three-strand Plait.

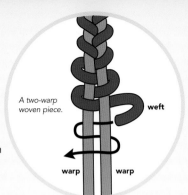

A two-warp woven piece.

weft

warp   warp

PLAIN
Easy rating ✔

Materials
Element 1 = 41 in (104 cm) = 1 strand of orange rattail

Element 2 = 12 in (30 cm) = 1 strand of orange rattail

Element 3 = 12 in (30 cm) = 1 strand of orange rattail

Method
Follow the instructions for Weaving with Two Warps (see page 68).

TWO COLORS
Easy rating ✔

Materials
Element 1 = 46 in (117 cm) = 1 strand of burgundy ruched knitting ribbon

Element 2 = 12 in (30 cm) = 1 strand of pink ruched knitting ribbon

Element 3 = 12 in (30 cm) = 1 strand of pink ruched knitting ribbon

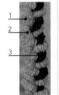

Method
Follow the instructions for Weaving with Two Warps (see page 68).

TWO COLORS
Easy rating ✔

Materials
Element 1 = 35 in (89 cm) = 1 strand of orange ruched knitting ribbon

Element 2 = 12 in (30 cm) = 1 strand of orange ruched knitting ribbon

Element 3 = 12 in (30 cm) = 1 strand of burgundy ruched knitting ribbon

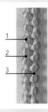

Method
Follow the instructions for Weaving with Two Warps (see page 68).

THREE COLORS
Easy rating ✔

Materials
Element 1 = 54 in (137 cm) = 1 strand of burgundy rattail

Element 2 = 12 in (30 cm) = 1 strand of pink rattail

Element 3 = 12 in (30 cm) = 1 strand of orange rattail

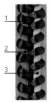

Method
Follow the instructions for Weaving with Two Warps (see page 68).

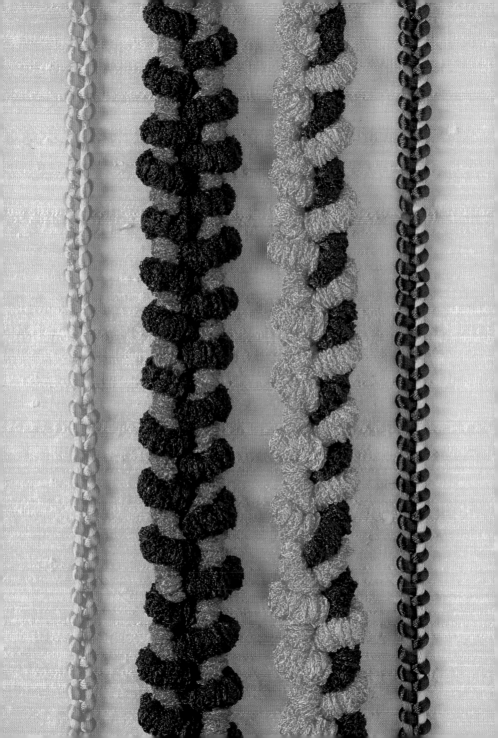

THICK WEFT

Materials

Element 1 = 46 in (117 cm) = 1 strand of orange crepe cord

Element 2 = 12 in (30 cm) = 1 strand of burgundy rattail

Element 3 = 12 in (30 cm) = 1 strand of burgundy rattail

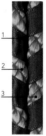

Method

Follow the instructions for Weaving with Two Warps (see page 68).

THICK WARPS

Materials

Element 1 = 99 in (251 cm) = 1 strand of 99 mm burgundy ribbon

Element 2 = 12 in (30 cm) = 1 strand of orange crepe cord

Element 3 = 12 in (30 cm) = 1 strand of orange crepe cord

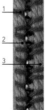

Method

Follow the instructions for Weaving with Two Warps (see page 68). Take care to keep the ribbon lying flat around the cord.

BEADED WEFT

Materials

Element 1 = 73 in (185 cm) = 1 strand of burgundy Double top cotton, threaded with 22 size 2° glass beads

Element 2 = 12 in (30 cm) = 4 strands of orange Chunky wool

Element 3 = 12 in (30 cm) = 4 strands of orange Chunky wool

Method

Follow the sequence for Weaving with Two Warps, Handheld (see page 68). Add a bead after every fourth repeat by making Step 2 (see page 68), then pushing a bead up the weft until it sits against the work. Continue with Step 3 so that the bead is trapped between the two warp threads.

BEADED WARP

Materials

Element 1 = 53 in (135 cm) = 1 strand of burgundy rattail

Element 2 = 12 in (30 cm) = 1 strand of pink rattail, threaded with 16 x size 2° glass beads

Element 3 = 12 in (30 cm) = 1 strand of pink rattail, threaded with 16 x size 2° glass beads

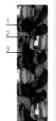

Method

Follow the sequence for Weaving with Two Warps, Handheld (see page 68). Work a sequence of Steps 2 to 5, then Steps 2 and 3. Push a bead up Element 2 until it sits against the work. Continue with Steps 4 and 5, trapping the bead in the work. Continue with a sequence of Steps 2 to 5, then push a bead up Element 3 until it sits against the work. Repeat the whole process again.

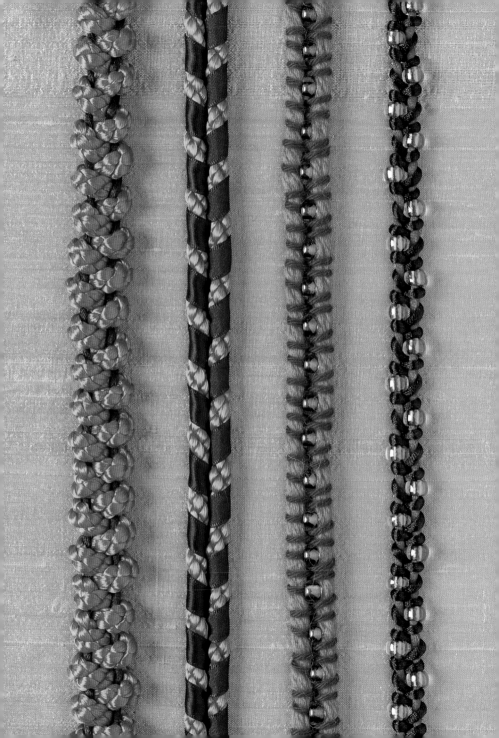

Two Warps, Weft-faced

These samples also have two warps, but they are distorted to produce a weft-faced result. This is achieved by keeping the two warp threads farther apart and pushing the weft firmly up over them so that the warp elements are completely hidden.

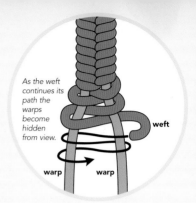

As the weft continues its path the warps become hidden from view.

weft

warp   **warp**

PLAIN

Materials

Element 1 = 73 in (185 cm) = 1 strand of burgundy rattail

Element 2 = 12 in (30 cm) = 1 strand of burgundy rattail. Element 2 is not visible

Element 3 = 12 in (30 cm) = 1 strand of burgundy rattail. Element 3 is not visible

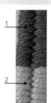

Method

Follow the instructions for Weaving with Two Warps (see page 68). Keep the weft pushed firmly up over the warps.

TWO COLORS
Easy rating ✔✔

Materials

Element 1 = 89 in (226 cm) = 1 strand of burgundy Double Top cotton

Element 2 = 12 in (30 cm) = 3 strands of burgundy Double Top cotton and 89 in (227 cm) =1 strand of pink Double Top cotton. Element 2 is not visible (except for one strand)

Element 3 = 12 in (30 cm) = 4 strands of burgundy Double Top cotton. Element 3 is not visible

Method

Work ten repeats of Weaving with Two Warps, Handheld, (see page 68). Now change the weft by swapping the burgundy weft with the long strand of pink cotton in Element 2. Work ten repeats of Weaving with Two Warps, Handheld before swapping the weft back into its original position.

TWO TEXTURES
Easy rating ✔✔

Materials

Element 1 = 44 in (112 cm) = 4 strands of burgundy knitting ribbon

Element 2 = 29 in (74 cm) = 16 strands of burgundy Kidsilk Haze mohair

Element 3 = 12 in (30 cm) = 4 strands of burgundy knitting ribbon. Element 3 is not visible

Method

Here the weft is changed by swapping all of Element 2 with Element 1. This is a section of Weaving with Two Warps, Handheld (see page 68). To swap the wefts, skip Step 2 before continuing as usual.

TWO COLORS AND BEADS
Easy rating ✔✔✔

Materials

Element 1 = 42 in (107 cm) = 4 strands of burgundy Glitter

Element 2 = 42 in (107 cm) = 4 strands of tan Glitter

Element 3 = 12 in (30 cm) = 4 strands of burgundy Glitter. Element 3 is not visible

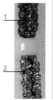

Method

Work a section of Weaving with Two Warps, Handheld (see page 68) using the burgundy Glitter as the weft. Add a pony bead by threading all of the elements through the bead using a fine crochet hook. Swap the weft by skipping the first Step 2, so that the tan Glitter becomes the weft. Work a section of weaving before adding another pony bead and swapping back to the burgundy weft.

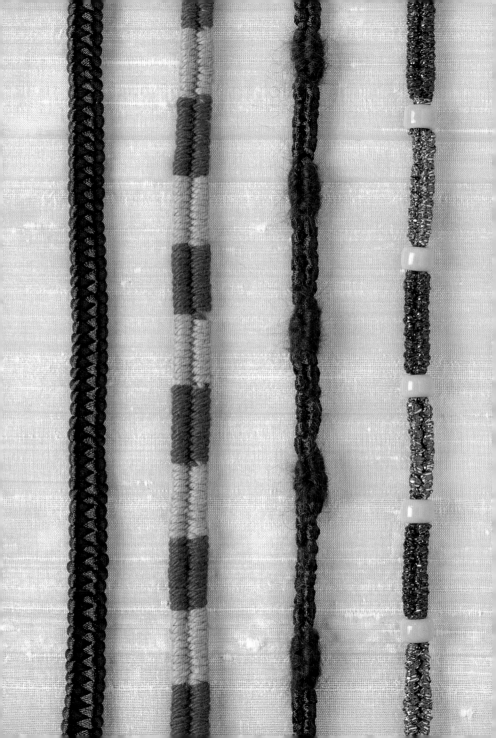

Three Warps

A slightly wider woven band is made by working with three warps (more than three warps can be used, making the weaving even wider). Samples using three warps have a tendency to twist because the weft turns around the outer elements in the same direction. The samples pictured have been flattened by carefully steaming the finished piece.

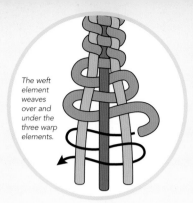

The weft element weaves over and under the three warp elements.

PLAIN

Easy rating ✔

Materials
Element 1 = 51 in (130 cm) = 1 strand of mauve rattail

Element 2 = 12 in (30 cm) = 1 strand of mauve rattail

Element 3 = 12 in (30 cm) = 1 strand of mauve rattail

Element 4 = 12 in (30 cm) = 1 strand of mauve rattail

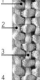

Method
Use the method for Weaving with Three Warps (see page 70).

TWO COLORS

Easy rating ✔

Materials
Element 1 = 57 in (145 cm) = 1 strand of purple Chunky wool

Element 2 = 12 in (30 cm) = 1 strand of mauve Chunky wool

Element 3 = 12 in (30 cm) = 1 strand of mauve Chunky wool

Element 4 = 12 in (30 cm) = 1 strand of mauve Chunky wool

Method
Use the method for Weaving with Three Warps (see page 70).

TWO COLORS

Easy rating ✔✔

Materials
Element 1 = 57 in (145 cm) = 4 strands of mauve knitting ribbon

Element 2 = 12 in (30 cm) = 4 strands of mauve knitting ribbon

Element 3 = 12 in (30 cm) = 4 strands of purple knitting ribbon

Element 4 = 12 in (30 cm) = 4 strands of mauve knitting ribbon

Method
Use the method for Weaving with Three Warps (see page 70). Take care to go under and over all of the strands in an element.

TWO COLORS

Easy rating ✔

Materials
Element 1 = 46 in (117 cm) = 1 strand of mauve ruched knitting ribbon

Element 2 = 12 in (30 cm) = 1 strand of purple ruched knitting ribbon

Element 3 = 12 in (30 cm) = 1 strand of mauve ruched knitting ribbon

Element 4 = 12 in (30 cm) = 1 strand of purple ruched knitting ribbon

Method
Use the method for Weaving with Three Warps (see page 70).

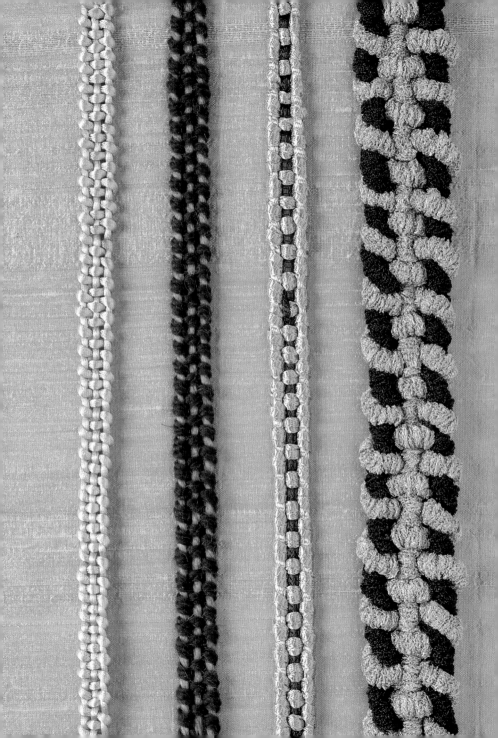

THREE COLORS

Easy rating ✔✔

Materials
Element 1 = 49 in (124 cm) = 4 strands of mauve knitting ribbon

Element 2 = 12 in (30 cm) = 4 strands of purple knitting ribbon

Element 3 = 12 in (30 cm) = 4 strands of mauve knitting ribbon

Element 4 = 12 in (30 cm) = 4 strands of blue knitting ribbon

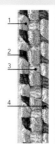

Method
Use the method for Weaving with Three Warps (see page 70). Take care to go under and over all of the strands in an element.

THREE COLORS

Easy rating ✔✔

Materials
Element 1 = 55 in (140 cm) = 4 strands of blue knitting ribbon

Element 2 = 12 in (30 cm) = 4 strands of blue knitting ribbon

Element 3 = 12 in (30 cm) = 4 strands of purple knitting ribbon

Element 4 = 12 in (30 cm) = 4 strands of mauve knitting ribbon

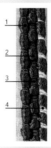
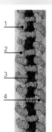

Method
Use the method for Weaving with Three Warps (see page 70). Take care to go under and over all of the strands in an element.

THREE COLORS

Easy rating ✔

Materials
Element 1 = 44 in (112 cm) = 1 strand of mid-blue ruched knitting ribbon

Element 2 = 12 in (30 cm) = 1 strand of mauve ruched knitting ribbon

Element 3 = 12 in (30 cm) = 1 strand of purple ruched knitting ribbon

Element 4 = 12 in (30 cm) = 1 strand of mauve ruched knitting ribbon

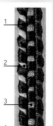

Method
Use the method for Weaving with Three Warps (see page 70).

FOUR COLORS

Easy rating ✔✔

Materials
Element 1 = 51 in (130 cm) = 8 strands of purple knitting ribbon

Element 2 = 12 in (30 cm) = 8 strands of light blue knitting ribbon

Element 3 = 12 in (30 cm) = 8 strands of mid-blue knitting ribbon

Element 4 = 12 in (30 cm) = 8 strands of dark blue knitting ribbon

Method
Use the method for Weaving with Three Warps (see page 70). Take care to go under and over all of the strands in an element.

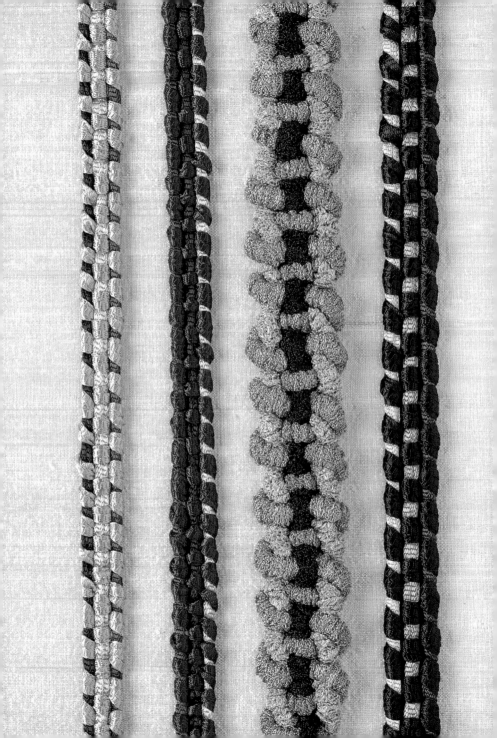

PLAIN

Materials

Element 1 = 257 in (653 cm) = 1 strand of blue Double Top cotton

Element 2 = 12 in (30 cm) = 4 strands of blue Double Top cotton

Element 3 = 12 in (30 cm) = 4 strands of blue Double Top cotton

Element 4 = 12 in (30 cm) = 4 strands of blue Double Top cotton

Elements 2, 3, and 4 are not visible

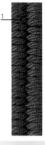

Method

Use the method for Weaving with Three Warps (see page 70). Keep the warp elements slightly apart and push the weft firmly up against the weaving.

RIBBON

Materials

Element 1 = 82 in (208 cm) = 1 strand of mauve knitting ribbon

Element 2 = 12 in (30 cm) = 1 strand of purple rattail

Element 3 = 12 in (30 cm) = 1 strand of 7 mm purple ribbon

Element 4 = 12 in (30 cm) = 1 strand of purple rattail

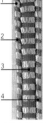

Method

Use the method for Weaving with Three Warps (see page 70). Keep both the central ribbon and the knitting ribbon lying flat.

WITH BEADS

Materials

Element 1 = 65 in (165 cm) = 1 strand of blue Russia braid

Element 2 = 12 in (30 cm) = 2 strands of mauve lacing cord

Element 3 = 12 in (30 cm) = 1 string of size 8° mauve rocaille beads

Element 4 = 12 in (30 cm) = 2 strands of mauve lacing cord

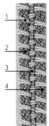

Method

Use the method for Weaving with Three Warps (see page 70). Make sure the pairs of lacing cords remain parallel to each other and keep the Russia braid lying flat.

WITH BEADS

Materials

Element 1 = 85 in (216 cm) = 1 strand of purple knitting ribbon

Element 2 = 12 in (30 cm) = 2 strands of purple knitting ribbon threaded with 66 x size 6° blue beads

Element 3 = 12 in (30 cm) = 1 strand of mauve lacing cord

Element 4 = 12 in (30 cm) = 2 strands of purple knitting ribbon threaded with 66 x size 6° blue beads

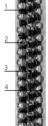

Method

Use the method for Weaving with Three Warps (see page 70). Make Step 2, then push a bead up Element 2 so that it sits against the edge of the weaving. Make Step 3, then add a bead from Element 4 so that it sits against the edge of the weaving.

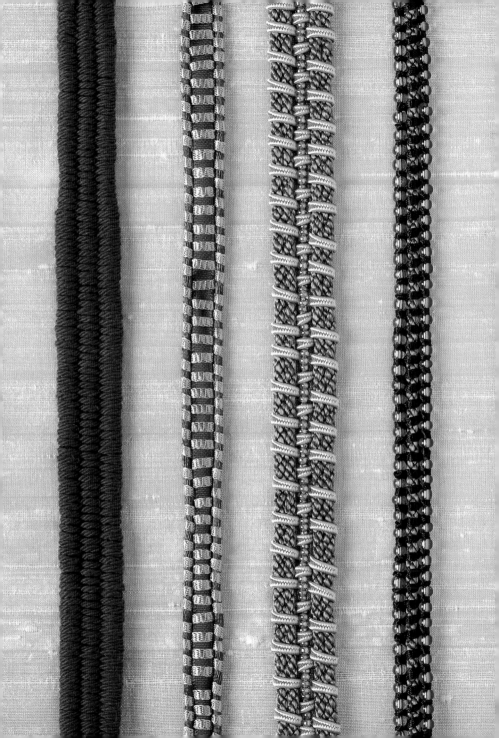

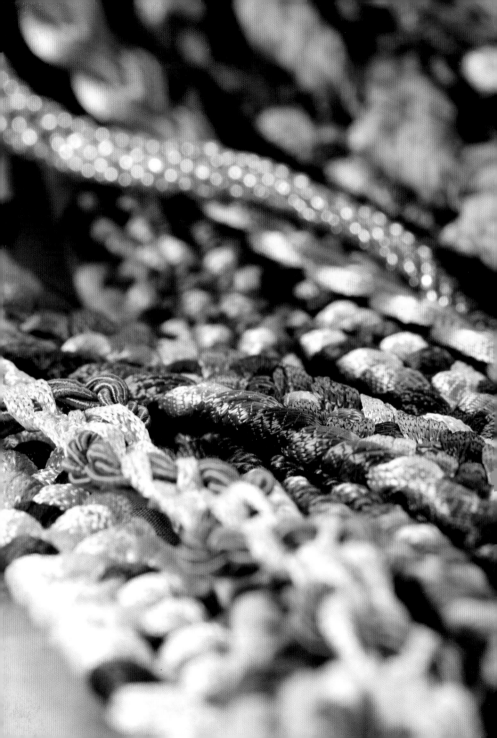

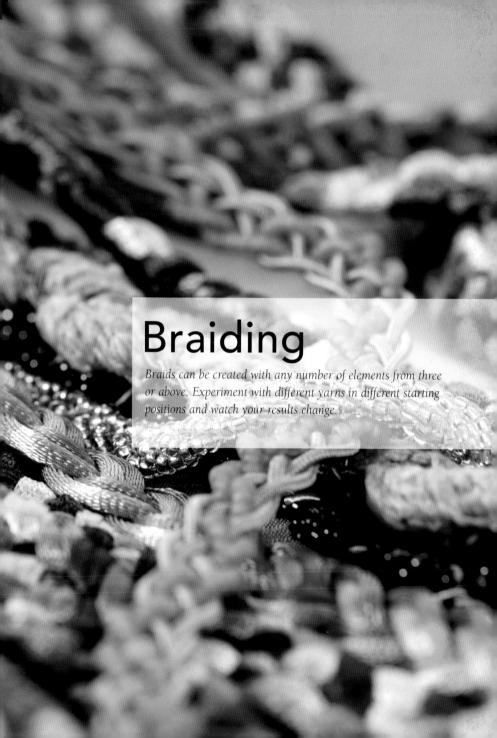

Braiding

Braids can be created with any number of elements from three or above. Experiment with different yarns in different starting positions and watch your results change.

Three-element Braid

The three-element braid is the most common braid structure, and it can be found all over the world. It has many names including the English Sinnet, Ordinary Sinnet, Flat Sinnet, Common Braid, Pigtail Braid, and Simple Plait.

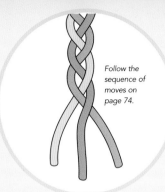

Follow the sequence of moves on page 74.

PLAIN

Easy rating

Materials
Element 1 = 14 in (36 cm) = 1 strand of green rattail

Element 2 = 14 in (36 cm) = 1 strand of green rattail

Element 3 = 14 in (36 cm) = 1 strand of green rattail

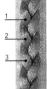

Method
Follow the instructions for Three-element Braid (see page 74).

TWO COLORS

Easy rating

Materials
Element 1 = 16 in (41 cm) = 6 strands of green Double Top cotton

Element 2 = 16 in (41 cm) = 6 strands of light green Double Top cotton

Element 3 = 16 in (41 cm) = 6 strands of light green Double Top cotton

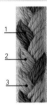

Method
Follow the instructions for Three-element Braid (see page 74).

THREE COLORS

Easy rating

Materials
Element 1 = 14 in (36 cm) = 1 strand of green gimp

Element 2 = 14 in (36 cm) = 1 strand of ocher gimp

Element 3 = 14 in (36 cm) = 1 strand of light green gimp

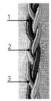

Method
Follow the instructions for Three-element Braid (see page 74).

THICK AND THIN

Easy rating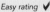

Materials
Element 1 = 15 in (38 cm) = 1 strand of ocher rattail

Element 2 = 12 in (30 cm) = 10 strands of green Double Top cotton

Element 3 = 15 in (38 cm) = 1 strand of ocher rattail

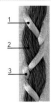

Method
Follow the instructions for Three-element Braid (see page 74). Work loosely, pulling Element 2 firmly so that it remains straight and in the center.

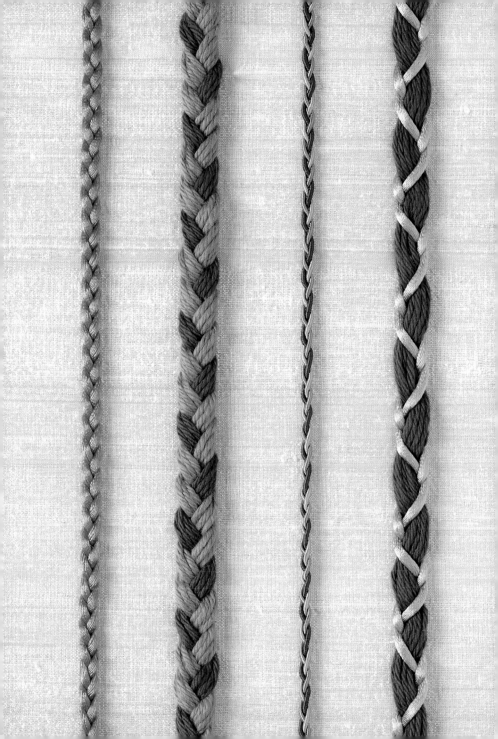

PAIRS PARALLEL

Easy rating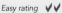

Materials

Element 1 = 15 in (38 cm) = 1 strand of green rattail and 1 strand of ocher rattail

Element 2 = 15 in (38 cm) = 1 strand of green rattail and 1 strand of ocher rattail

Element 3 = 15 in (38 cm) = 1 strand of green rattail and 1 strand of ocher rattail

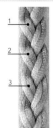

Method

Start each element with the green on the right-hand side. Follow the instructions for Three-element Braid (see page 74), keeping the strands of each element parallel, so that the green remains on the right-hand side of the ocher strand.

PAIRS FOLDED

Easy rating

Materials

Element 1 = 15 in (38 cm) = 1 strand of green rattail and 1 strand of ocher rattail

Element 2 = 15 in (38 cm) = 1 strand of green rattail and 1 strand of ocher rattail

Element 3 = 15 in (38 cm) = 1 strand of green rattail and 1 strand of ocher rattail

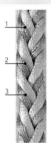

Method

Follow the instructions for Three-element Braid (see page 74), folding the elements so that the ocher strand is always above the green strand.

RIBBON

Easy rating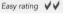

Materials

Element 1 = 16 in (41 cm) = 1 strand of 15 mm green ribbon

Element 2 = 16 in (41 cm) = 1 strand of 15 mm green ribbon

Element 3 = 16 in (41 cm) = 1 strand of 15 mm green ribbon

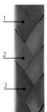

Method

Follow the instructions for Three-element Braid (see page 74), folding over the ribbon at the edges. Iron the finished braid to make neat creases at the edge.

BEADED WARP

Easy rating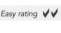

Materials

Element 1 = 16 in (41 cm) = 1 strand of 15 mm green ribbon

Element 2 = 16 in (41 cm) = 1 strand of 15 mm ocher ribbon

Element 3 = 16 in (41 cm) = 1 strand of 15 mm ocher ribbon

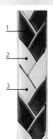

Method

Start each element with the green ribbon on top of the ocher ribbon. Follow the instructions for Three-element Braid (see page 74), folding over the ribbon at the edges, so that the reverse side is visible. Iron the finished braid to make neat creases at the edge.

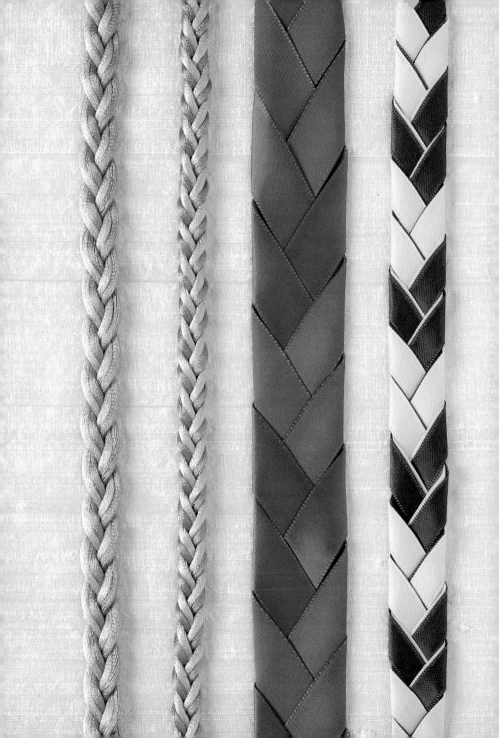

GLITTER AND GIMP
Easy rating ✔

Materials
Element 1 = 19 in (48 cm) = 20 strands of green Glitter

Element 2 = 13 in (33 cm) = 1 strand of ocher gimp

Element 3 = 13 in (33 cm) = 1 strand of ocher gimp

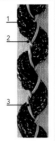

Method
Follow the instructions for Three-element Braid (see page 74).

DISTORTED
Easy rating ✔

Materials
Element 1 = 12 in (30 cm) = 1 strand of green Russia braid

Element 2 = 45 in (114 cm) = 8 strands of green gimp

Element 3 = 49 in (124 cm) = 4 strands of green Glitter

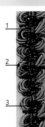

Method
Follow the instructions for Three-element Braid (see page 74). Work loosely and evenly, keeping the Russia braid lying flat without any folds in it. After every few sequences, distort the braid by pulling on the Russia braid element and sliding the gimp and Glitter up toward the fixed point.

WITH BEADS
Easy rating ✔

Materials
Element 1 = 17 in (43 cm) = 1 string of gold size 11° rocaille beads

Element 2 = 17 in (43 cm) = 16 strands of ocher No 5 pearl cotton

Element 3 = 17 in (43 cm) = 6 strands of green knitting ribbon

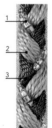

Method
Follow the instructions for Three-element Braid (see page 74).

WITH BEADS
Easy rating ✔

Materials
Element 1 = 12 in (30 cm) = 1 string of malachite chip beads

Element 2 = 13 in (33 cm) = 3 strands of ocher gimp

Element 3 = 13 in (33 cm) = 3 strands of ocher gimp

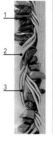

Method
Follow the instructions for Three-element Braid (see page 74), working loosely to allow the gimp to fall over and between the beads.

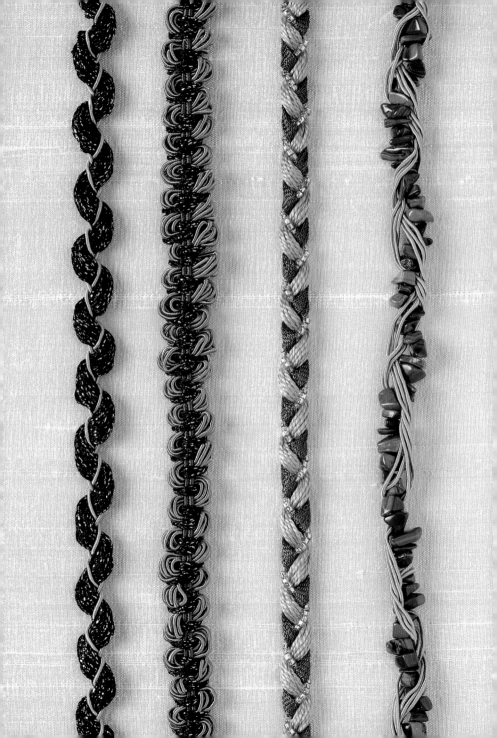

Four-element Flat Braid

This braid is a little wider and has three ridges. As both of the outer ridges slant in the same direction, it can put a slight twist into the finished result. The braid can be straightened by carefully steaming it.

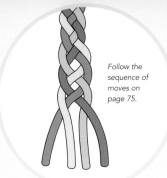

Follow the sequence of moves on page 75.

PLAIN

Easy rating ✔

Materials

Element 1 =15 in (38 cm) = 1 strand of ocher rattail

Element 2 =15 in (38 cm) = 1 strand of ocher rattail

Element 3 =15 in (38 cm) = 1 strand of ocher rattail

Element 4 =15 in (38 cm) = 1 strand of ocher rattail

Method

Follow the method for Four-element Flat Braid (see page 75).

TWO COLORS 1:3

Easy rating ✔

Materials

Element 1 = 18 in (46 cm) = 8 strands of yellow knitting ribbon

Element 2 = 18 in (46 cm) = 8 strands of red knitting ribbon

Element 3 = 18 in (46 cm) = 8 strands of red knitting ribbon

Element 4 = 18 in (46 cm) = 8 strands of red knitting ribbon

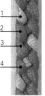

Method

Follow the method for Four-element Flat Braid (see page 75). Take care to keep all the strands together for each element.

TWO COLORS 2:2

Easy rating ✔

Materials

Element 1 = 17 in (43 cm) = 8 strands of red Glitter

Element 2 = 17 in (43 cm) = 8 strands of ocher Glitter

Element 3 = 17 in (43 cm) = 8 strands of ocher Glitter

Element 4 = 17 in (43 cm) = 8 strands of red Glitter

Method

Follow the method for Four-element Flat Braid (see page 75). Take care to keep all the strands together for each element.

TWO COLORS 2:2

Easy rating ✔

Materials

Element 1 = 17 in (43 cm) = 8 strands of ocher knitting ribbon

Element 2 = 17 in (43 cm) = 8 strands of ocher knitting ribbon

Element 3 = 17 in (43 cm) = 8 strands of red knitting ribbon

Element 4 = 17 in (43 cm) = 8 strands of red knitting ribbon

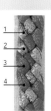

Method

Follow the method for Four-element Flat Braid (see page 75). Take care to keep all the strands together for each element.

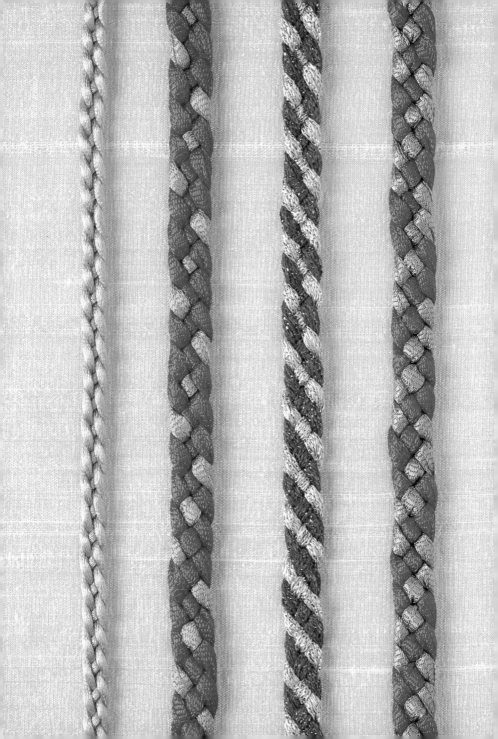

THREE COLORS 1:1:2

Easy rating

Materials

Element 1 = 16 in (41 cm) = 2 strands of brown Double Top wool

Element 2 = 16 in (41 cm) = 2 strands of red Double Top wool

Element 3 = 16 in (41 cm) = 2 strands of orange Double Top wool

Element 4 = 16 in (41 cm) = 2 strands of brown Double Top wool

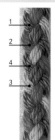

Method

Follow the method for Four-element Flat Braid (see page 75). Keep the two strands in each element lying parallel at all times

THREE COLORS 1:1:2

Easy rating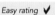

Materials

Element 1 = 17 in (43 cm) = 10 strands of red Glitter

Element 2 = 17 in (43 cm) = 10 strands of red Glitter

Element 3 = 17 in (43 cm) = 10 strands of brown Glitter

Element 4 = 17 in (43 cm) = 10 strands of yellow Glitter

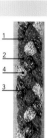

Method

Follow the method for Four-element Flat Braid (see page 75).

FOUR COLORS

Easy rating

Materials

Element 1 = 17 in (43 cm) = 8 strands of red knitting ribbon

Element 2 = 17 in (43 cm) = 8 strands of brown knitting ribbon

Element 3 = 17 in (43 cm) = 8 strands of ocher knitting ribbon

Element 4 = 17 in (43 cm) = 8 strands of yellow knitting ribbon

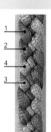

Method

Follow the instructions for Four-element Flat Braid (see page 75), taking care to keep all the strands together for each element.

TWO TEXTURES

Easy rating

Materials

Element 1 = 21 in (53 cm) = 2 strands of Ribbon Twist wool

Element 2 = 21 in (53 cm) = 2 strands of Ribbon Twist wool

Element 3 = 15 in (38 cm) = 1 strand of ocher rattail

Element 4 = 15 in (38 cm) = 1 strand of ocher rattail

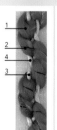

Method

Follow the instructions for Four-element Flat Braid (see page 75). Pull Elements 3 and 4 slightly more firmly to give the scallop edge.

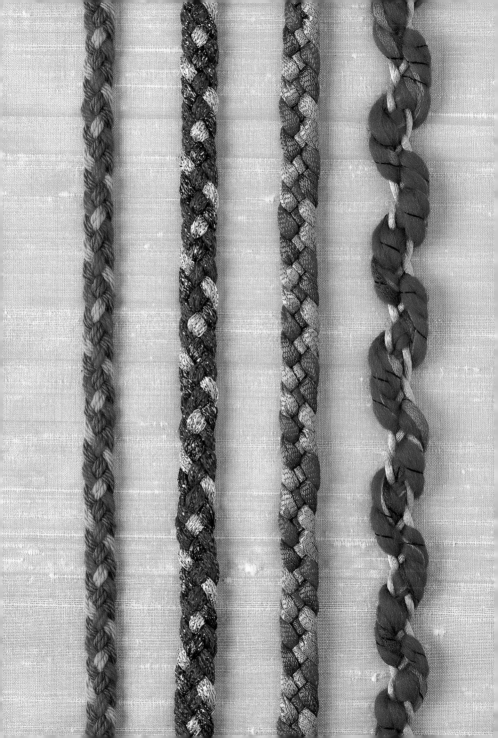

TWO TEXTURES

Easy rating ✔

Materials
Element 1 = 13 in (33 cm) = 1 strand of ruched knitting ribbon

Element 2 = 17 in (43 cm) = 1 strand of ocher rattail

Element 3 = 17 in (43 cm) = 1 strand of ocher rattail

Element 4 = 17 in (43 cm) = 1 strand of ocher rattail

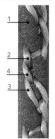

Method
Follow the instructions for Four-element Flat Braid (see page 75).

WITH BEADS

Easy rating ✔ ✔

Materials
Element 1 = 21 in (53 cm) = 4 strands of Glitter, threaded with 27 4-mm red glass beads

Element 2 = 21 in (53 cm) = 4 strands of Glitter, threaded with 27 4-mm red glass beads

Element 3 = 21 in (53 cm) = 4 strands of Glitter, threaded with 27 4-mm red glass beads

Element 4 = 21 in (53 cm) = 4 strands of Glitter, threaded with 27 4-mm red glass beads

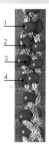

Method
Follow the instructions for Four-element Flat Braid (see page 75). Before every Step 2, push a bead up from the element on the leftmost and rightmost position. Keep these beads close to the work, making Steps 2 and 3 under them. Allow the finished braid to retain the twist.

WITH BEADS

Easy rating ✔

Materials
Element 1 = 15 in (38 cm) = 1 string of yellow size 11° rocaille beads

Element 2 = 17 in (43 cm) = 1 strand of ocher knitting ribbon

Element 3 = 17 in (43 cm) = 8 strands of ocher knitting ribbon

Element 4 = 15 in (38 cm) = 1 string of yellow size 11° rocaille beads

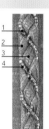

Method
Follow the instructions for Four-element Flat Braid (see page 75).

WITH BEADS

Easy rating ✔ ✔

Materials
Element 1 = 13 in (33 cm) = 1 strand of red Japanese braid

Element 2 = 17 in (43 cm) = 1 strand of ocher Japanese braid threaded with 8 5-mm metallic beads

Element 3 = 17 in (43 cm) = 1 strand of ocher Japanese braid threaded with 8 5-mm metallic beads

Element 4 = 13 in (33 cm) = 1 strand of red Japanese braid

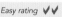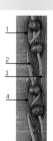

Method
Follow the instructions for Four-element Flat Braid (see page 75). Work a repeat of Steps 2 to 4. Then make another Step 2 and 3 before pushing up a bead from the element in the center-left position. Make Step 4 and push up another bead from the center-right position (it will be the same element). Repeat this procedure, keeping the tension loose so that the elements form a lattice structure.

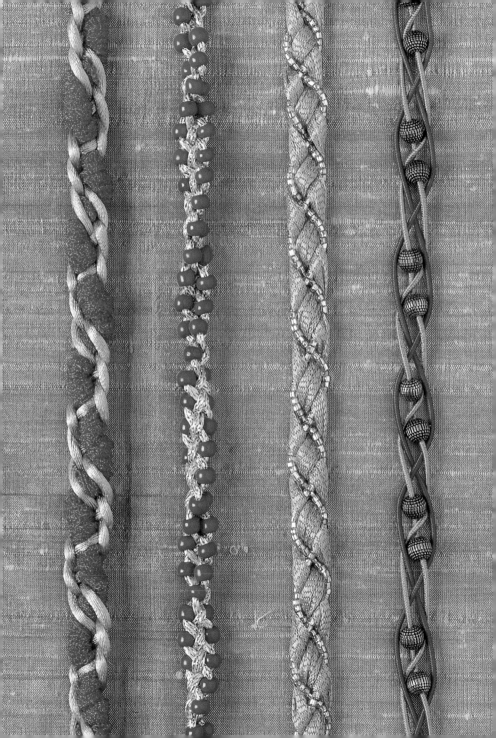

Four-element Round Braid

This is another braid worked with four elements. However, this produces a three-dimensional braid with four sides. It is sometimes called square, though more often it is referred to as round, proceeded by the word braid, sinnet, or plait.

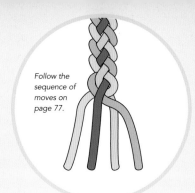

Follow the sequence of moves on page 77.

PLAIN

Easy rating ✔

Materials
Element 1 = 15 in (38 cm) = 1 strand of purple rattail

Element 2 = 15 in (38 cm) = 1 strand of purple rattail

Element 3 = 15 in (38 cm) = 1 strand of purple rattail

Element 4 = 15 in (38 cm) = 1 strand of purple rattail

Method
Follow the method for Four-element Round Braid (see page 77).

TWO COLORS 3:1

Easy rating ✔

Materials
Element 1 = 15 in (38 cm) = 2 strands of lilac Chunky wool

Element 2 = 15 in (38 cm) = 2 strands of purple Chunky wool

Element 3 = 15 in (38 cm) = 2 strands of purple Chunky wool

Element 4 = 15 in (38 cm) = 2 strands of purple Chunky wool

Method
Follow the method for Four-element Round Braid (see page 77).

TWO COLORS 2:2

Easy rating ✔

Materials
Element 1 = 18 in (46 cm) = 8 strands of pink knitting ribbon

Element 2 = 18 in (46 cm) = 8 strands of purple knitting ribbon

Element 3 = 18 in (46 cm) = 8 strands of pink knitting ribbon

Element 4 = 18 in (46 cm) = 8 strands of purple knitting ribbon

Method
Follow the method for Four-element Round Braid (see page 77).

TWO COLORS 2:2

Easy rating ✔

Materials
Element 1 = 16 in (41 cm) = 8 strands of purple knitting ribbon

Element 2 = 16 in (41 cm) = 8 strands of purple knitting ribbon

Element 3 = 16 in (41 cm) = 8 strands of lilac knitting ribbon

Element 4 = 16 in (41 cm) = 8 strands of lilac knitting ribbon

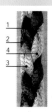

Method
Follow the method for Four-element Round Braid (see page 77).

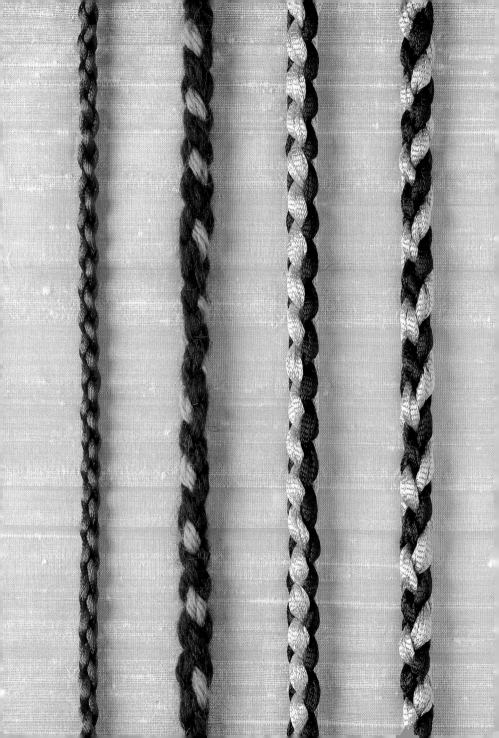

THREE COLORS

Materials

Element 1 = 19 in (48 cm) = 8 strands of lilac knitting ribbon

Element 2 = 19 in (48 cm) = 8 strands of pink knitting ribbon

Element 3 = 19 in (48 cm) = 8 strands of purple knitting ribbon

Element 4 = 19 in (48 cm) = 8 strands of purple knitting ribbon

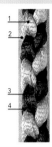

Method

Follow the method for Four-element Round Braid (see page 77).

THREE COLORS

Easy rating ✔

Materials

Element 1 = 16 in (41 cm) = 8 strands of purple knitting ribbon

Element 2 = 16 in (41 cm) = 8 strands of lilac knitting ribbon

Element 3 = 16 in (41 cm) = 8 strands of purple knitting ribbon

Element 4 = 16 in (41 cm) = 8 strands of pink knitting ribbon

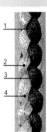

Method

Follow the method for Four-element Round Braid (see page 77).

FOUR COLORS

Easy rating ✔

Materials

Element 1 = 18 in (46 cm) = 4 strands of pink Double Top cotton

Element 2 = 18 in (46 cm) = 4 strands of lilac Double Top cotton

Element 3 = 18 in (46 cm) = 4 strands of dark pink Double Top cotton

Element 4 = 18 in (46 cm) = 4 strands of purple Double Top cotton

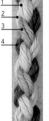

Method

Follow the method for Four-element Round Braid (see page 77).

TWO THICKNESSES

Easy rating ✔✔

Materials

Element 1 = 17 in (43 cm) = 2 strands of purple Chunky wool

Element 2 = 17 in (43 cm) = 2 strands of purple Chunky wool

Element 3 = 17 in (43 cm) = 2 strands of purple Chunky wool

Element 4 = 17 in (43 cm) = 6 strands of lilac Chunky wool

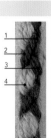

Method

Follow the method for Four-element Round Braid (see page 77).

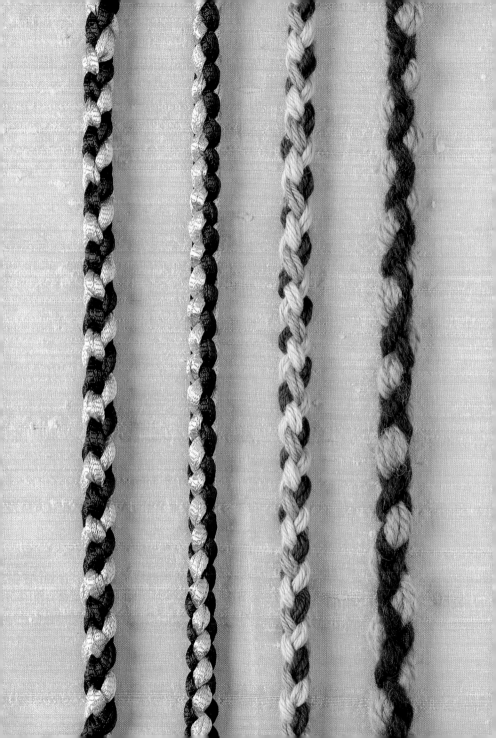

TWO TEXTURES

Easy rating ✔

Materials

Element 1 = 16 in (41 cm) = 2 strands of purple gimp

Element 2 = 16 in (41 cm) = 2 strands of purple gimp

Element 3 = 19 in (48 cm) = 10 strands of purple Calmer cotton

Element 4 = 19 in (48 cm) = 10 strands of purple Calmer cotton

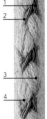

Method

Follow the method for Four-element Round Braid (see page 77), pulling firmly on the gimp.

TWO TEXTURES

Easy rating ✔✔

Materials

Element 1 = 16 in (41 cm) = 1 strand of lilac lacing cord

Element 2 = 18 in (46 cm) = 1 strand of pink Russia braid

Element 3 = 16 in (41 cm) = 1 strand of lilac lacing cord

Element 4 = 18 in (46 cm) = 1 strand of pink Russia braid

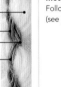

Method

Follow the method for Four-element Round Braid (see page 77). Take care to fold the Russia braid around the cord so that it lies flat against it.

TWO TEXTURES

Easy rating ✔

Materials

Element 1 = 19 in (48 cm) = 16 strands of lilac Baby Soft wool

Element 2 = 15 in (38 cm) = 2 strands of purple gimp

Element 3 = 15 in (38 cm) = 2 strands of purple gimp

Element 4 = 15 in (38 cm) = 2 strands of purple gimp

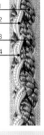

Method

Follow the method for Four-element Round Braid (see page 77).

TWO TEXTURES

Easy rating ✔✔

Materials

Element 1 = 13 in (33 cm) = 1 strand of pink Japanese braid

Element 2 = 14 in (36 cm) = 1 purple four-element flat braid (see page 202)

Element 3 = 13 in (33 cm) = 1 strand of pink Japanese braid

Element 4 = 14 in (36 cm) = 1 purple four-element flat braid (see page 202)

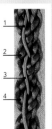

Method

Follow the method for Four-element Round Braid (see page 77). Take care to keep Elements 3 and 4 flat at all times.

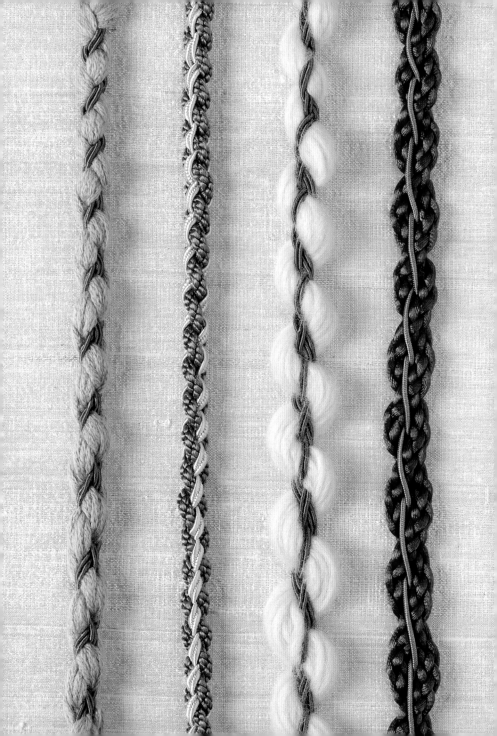

Four-element Chain-link Braid

This is a delightful little four-element braid. The elements follow slightly different paths, with one pair working more frequently than the other. This results in the chain-link effect.

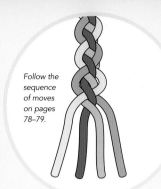

Follow the sequence of moves on pages 78–79.

PLAIN

Easy rating ✔✔

Materials
Element 1 = 14 in (36 cm) = 1 strand of ocher rattail

Element 2 = 14 in (36 cm) = 1 strand of ocher rattail

Element 3 = 14 in (36 cm) = 1 strand of ocher rattail

Element 4 = 14 in (36 cm) = 1 strand of ocher rattail

Method
Follow the method for Four-element Chain-link Braid (see page 78).

TWO COLORS 3:1

Easy rating ✔✔

Materials
Element 1 = 16 in (41 cm) = 20 strands of cream No 5 pearl cotton

Element 2 = 16 in (41 cm) = 20 strands of gold No 5 pearl cotton

Element 3 = 16 in (41 cm) = 20 strands of gold No 5 pearl cotton

Element 4 = 16 in (41 cm) = 20 strands of gold No 5 pearl cotton

Method
Follow the method for Four-element Chain-link Braid (see page 78).

TWO COLORS 3:1

Easy rating ✔✔

Materials
Element 1 = 16 in (41 cm) = 20 strands of gold No 5 pearl cotton

Element 2 = 16 in (41 cm) = 20 strands of cream No 5 pearl cotton

Element 3 = 16 in (41 cm) = 20 strands of gold No 5 pearl cotton

Element 4 = 16 in (41 cm) = 20 strands of gold No 5 pearl cotton

Method
Follow the method for Four-element Chain-link Braid (see page 78).

TWO COLORS 2:2

Easy rating ✔✔

Materials
Element 1 = 16 in (41 cm) = 10 strands of yellow No 5 pearl cotton

Element 2 = 16 in (41 cm) = 10 strands of gold No 5 pearl cotton

Element 3 = 16 in (41 cm) = 10 strands of yellow No 5 pearl cotton

Element 4 = 16 in (41 cm) = 10 strands of gold No 5 pearl cotton

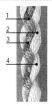

Method
Follow the method for Four-element Chain-link Braid (see page 78).

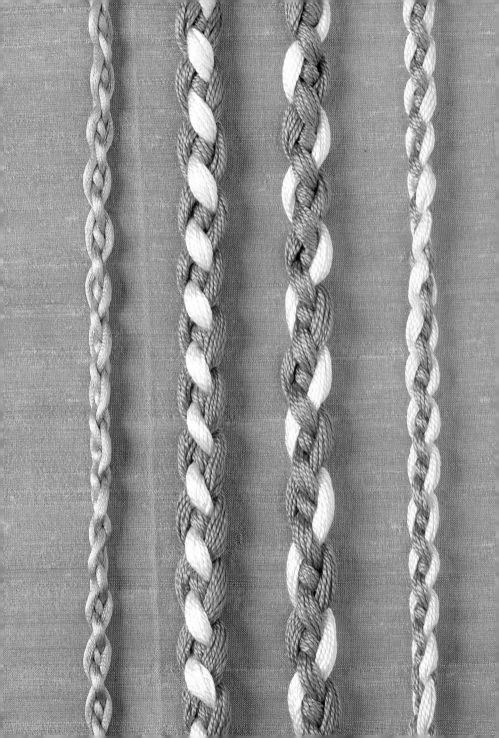

TWO COLORS 2:2

Easy rating ✔✔

Materials

Element 1 = 16 in (41 cm) = 10 strands of gold No 5 pearl cotton

Element 2 = 16 in (41 cm) = 10 strands of gold No 5 pearl cotton

Element 3 = 16 in (41 cm) = 10 strands of yellow No 5 pearl cotton

Element 4 = 16 in (41 cm) = 10 strands of yellow No 5 pearl cotton

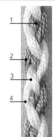

Method

Follow the method for Four-element Chain-link Braid (see page 78).

THREE COLORS 1:1:2

Easy rating ✔✔

Materials

Element 1 = 18 in (46 cm) = 16 strands of dark gold Glitter

Element 2 = 18 in (46 cm) = 16 strands of light gold Glitter

Element 3 = 18 in (46 cm) = 16 strands of mid gold Glitter

Element 4 = 18 in (46 cm) = 16 strands of light gold Glitter

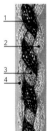

Method

Follow the method for Four-element Chain-link Braid (see page 78).

THREE COLORS 1:1:2

Easy rating ✔✔

Materials

Element 1 =16 in (41 cm) = 10 strands of cream No 5 pearl cotton

Element 2 = 16 in (41 cm) = 10 strands of burgundy No 5 pearl cotton

Element 3 =16 in (41 cm) = 10 strands of cream No 5 pearl cotton

Element 4 = 16 in (41 cm) = 10 strands of gold No 5 pearl cotton

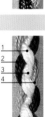

Method

Follow the method for Four-element Chain-link Braid (see page 78).

FOUR COLORS

Easy rating ✔✔

Materials

Element 1 = 17 in (43 cm) = 16 strands of burgundy No 5 pearl cotton

Element 2 = 17 in (43 cm) = 16 strands of gold No 5 pearl cotton

Element 3 = 17 in (43 cm) = 16 strands of ocher No 5 pearl cotton

Element 4 = 17 in (43 cm) = 16 strands of yellow No 5 pearl cotton

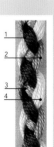

Method

Follow the method for Four-element Chain-link Braid (see page 78).

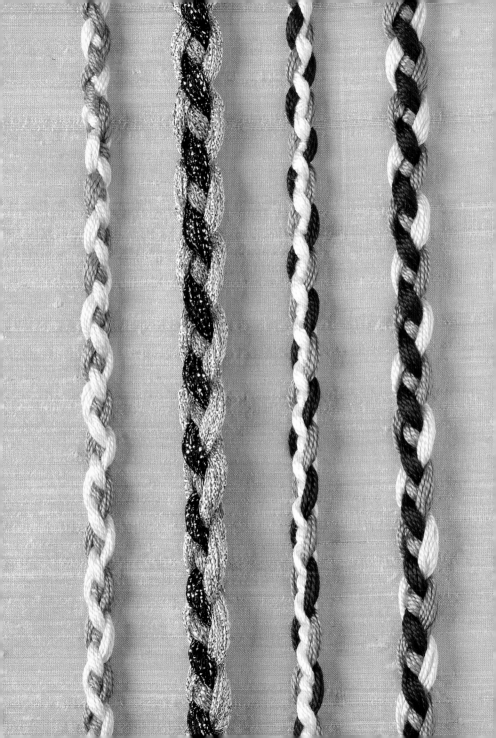

DIFFERENT TEXTURES

Easy rating ✔✔✔

Materials

Element 1 = 16 in (41 cm) = 1 strand of ocher Russia braid

Element 2 = 16 in (41 cm) = 1 strand of gold ruched knitting ribbon

Element 3 = 16 in (41 cm) = 1 strand of ocher Russia braid

Element 4 = 16 in (41 cm) = 1 strand of ocher ruched knitting ribbon

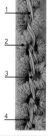

Method

Follow the method for "Four-element Chain-link" Braid (see page 78), keeping Elements 2 and 4 slightly loose.

DIFFERENT TEXTURES

Easy rating ✔✔

Materials

Element 1 = 15 in (38 cm) = 6 strands of yellow gimp

Element 2 = 15 in (38 cm) = 16 strands of gold No 5 pearl cotton

Element 3 = 15 in (38 cm) = 6 strands of Tinsel

Element 4 = 15 in (38 cm) = 16 strands of gold No 5 pearl cotton

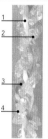

Method

Follow the method for "Four-element Chain-link" Braid (see page 78)

WITH BEADS

Easy rating ✔✔

Materials

Element 1 = 15 in (38 cm) = 1 strand of cream rattail

Element 2 = 16 in (41 cm) = 1 strand of citrine chips

Element 3 = 15 in (38 cm) = 1 strand of ocher rattail

Element 4 = 16 in (41 cm) = 1 strand of citrine chips

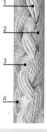

Method

Follow the method for "Four-element Chain-link" Braid (see page 78).

WITH BEADS

Easy rating ✔✔✔

Materials

Element 1 = 16 in (41 cm) = 6 strands of ocher knitting ribbon

Element 2 = 16 in (41 cm) = 1 strand of yellow gimp, threaded with 66 4-mm glass beads

Element 3 = 16 in (41 cm) = 6 strands of yellow knitting ribbon

Element 4 = 16 in (41 cm) = 1 strand of yellow gimp, threaded with 66 4-mm glass beads.

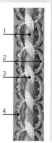

Method

Follow the method for "Four-element Chain-link" Braid (see page 78), working repeats of the following instructions. Make Steps 2 and 3, making sure that these are firmly tightened. Then push three beads up Element 2 and 4 until they are sitting against the braid. Make Steps 4 and 5. Do not pull these too tight as the beads need to sit in a slight curve away from the braid.

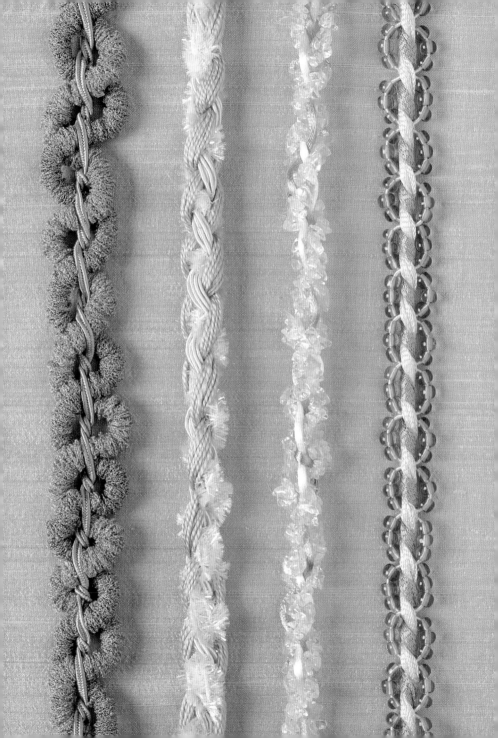

Five-element, Two-ridge Braid

This is an extension of the common three-element braid, where two moves are made, taking the outer element to the opposite center. The result is a two-ridge braid like the three-element braid. However, it is fuller and has the ability to produce more patterns than its smaller counterpart. It is often called a Russia, or Soutache braid.

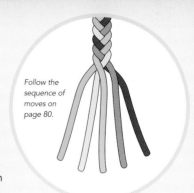

Follow the sequence of moves on page 80.

PLAIN

Easy rating ✔

Materials
Element 1 = 15 in (38 cm) = 1 strand of gray rattail

Element 2 = 15 in (38 cm) = 1 strand of gray rattail

Element 3 = 15 in (38 cm) = 1 strand of gray rattail

Element 4 = 15 in (38 cm) = 1 strand of gray rattail

Element 5 = 15 in (38 cm) = 1 strand of gray rattail

Method
Follow the method for Five-element, Two-ridge Braid (see page 80).

TWO COLORS 1:4

Easy rating ✔

Materials
Element 1 = 15 in (38 cm) = 10 strands of pink No 5 pearl cotton
Element 2 = 15 in (38 cm) = 10 strands of gray No 5 pearl cotton
Element 3 = 15 in (38 cm) = 10 strands of gray No 5 pearl cotton
Element 4 = 15 in (38 cm) = 10 strands of gray No 5 pearl cotton
Element 5 = 15 in (38 cm) = 10 strands of gray No 5 pearl cotton

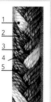

Method
Follow the method for Five-element, Two-ridge Braid (see page 80). Take care to keep all the strands together for each element.

TWO COLORS 2:3

Easy rating ✔✔

Materials
Element 1 = 15 in (38 cm) = 10 strands of light gray No 5 pearl cotton
Element 2 = 15 in (38 cm) = 10 strands of light gray No 5 pearl cotton
Element 3 = 15 in (38 cm) = 10 strands of light gray No 5 pearl cotton
Element 4 = 15 in (38 cm) = 10 strands of gray No 5 pearl cotton
Element 5 = 15 in (38 cm) = 10 strands of gray No 5 pearl cotton

Method
Follow the method for Five-element, Two-ridge Braid (see page 80). Take care to keep all the strands together for each element.

TWO COLORS 2:3

Easy rating ✔✔

Materials
Element 1 = 15 in (38 cm) = 10 strands of gray No 5 pearl cotton
Element 2 = 15 in (38 cm) = 10 strands of pink No 5 pearl cotton
Element 3 = 15 in (38 cm) = 10 strands of pink No 5 pearl cotton
Element 4 = 15 in (38 cm) = 10 strands of pink No 5 pearl cotton
Element 5 = 15 in (38 cm) = 10 strands of gray No 5 pearl cotton

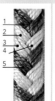

Method
Follow the method for Five-element, Two-ridge Braid (see page 80). Take care to keep all the strands together for each element.

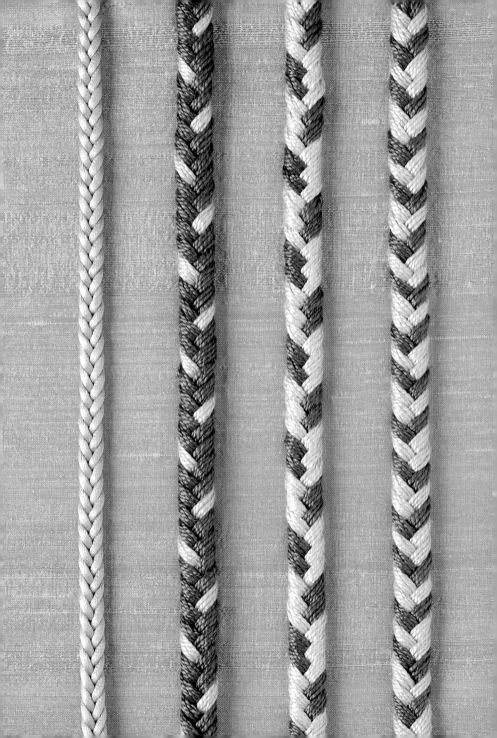

THREE COLORS 1:1:3

Easy rating

Materials

Element 1 = 15 in (38 cm) = 1 strand of gray rattail

Element 2 = 15 in (38 cm) = 1 strand of pink rattail

Element 3 = 15 in (38 cm) = 1 strand of pale pink rattail

Element 4 = 15 in (38 cm) = 1 strand of pink rattail

Element 5 = 15 in (38 cm) = 1 strand of pink rattail

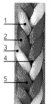

Method

Follow the method for Five-element, Two-ridge Braid (see page 80).

THREE COLORS 1:1:3

Easy rating

Materials

Element 1 = 15 in (38 cm) = 1 strand of light pink rattail

Element 2 = 15 in (38 cm) = 1 strand of pink rattail

Element 3 = 15 in (38 cm) = 1 strand of gray rattail

Element 4 = 15 in (38 cm) = 1 strand of gray rattail

Element 5 = 15 in (38 cm) = 1 strand of gray rattail

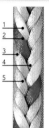

Method

Follow the method for Five-element, Two-ridge Braid (see page 80).

THREE COLORS 1:2:2

Easy rating

Materials

Element 1 = 15 in (38 cm) = 4 strands of purple Double Top cotton

Element 2 = 15 in (38 cm) = 4 strands of pink Double Top cotton

Element 3 = 15 in (38 cm) = 4 strands of purple Double Top cotton

Element 4 = 15 in (38 cm) = 4 strands of lilac Double Top cotton

Element 5 = 15 in (38 cm) = 4 strands of pink Double Top cotton

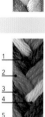

Method

Follow the method for Five-element, Two-ridge Braid (see page 80). Take care to keep all the strands together for each element.

THREE COLORS 1:2:2

Easy rating

Materials

Element 1 = 15 in (38 cm) = 10 strands of gray No 5 pearl cotton

Element 2 = 15 in (38 cm) = 10 strands of pink No 5 pearl cotton

Element 3 = 15 in (38 cm) = 10 strands of gray No 5 pearl cotton

Element 4 = 15 in (38 cm) = 10 strands of light gray No 5 pearl cotton

Element 5 = 15 in (38 cm) = 10 strands of light gray No 5 pearl cotton

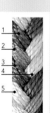

Method

Follow the method for Five-element, Two-ridge Braid (see page 80). Take care to keep all the strands together for each element.

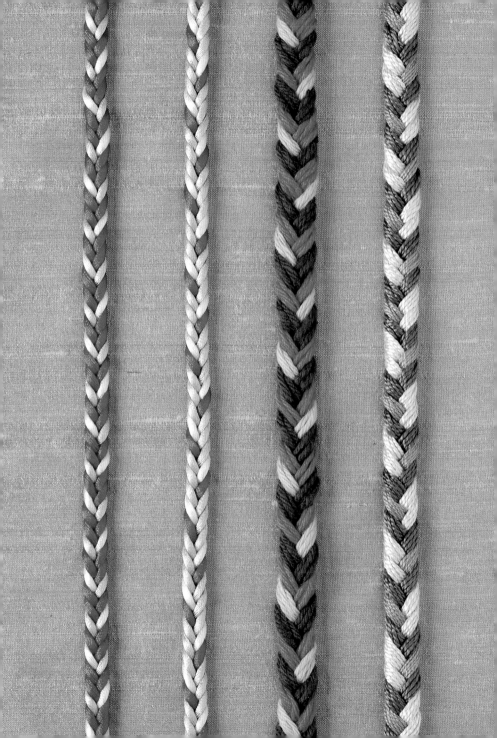

THREE COLORS 1:2:2

Easy rating ✔✔

Materials

Element 1 = 17 in (43 cm) = 6 strands of pink knitting ribbon

Element 2 = 17 in (43 cm) = 6 strands of gray knitting ribbon

Element 3 = 17 in (43 cm) = 6 strands of gray knitting ribbon

Element 4 = 17 in (43 cm) = 6 strands of mauve knitting ribbon

Element 5 = 17 in (43 cm) = 6 strands of mauve knitting ribbon

Method

Follow the method for Five-element, Two-ridge Braid (see page 80). Take care to keep all the strands together for each element.

FOUR COLORS 1:1:1:2

Easy rating ✔✔

Materials

Element 1 = 16 in (41 cm) = 6 strands of purple Double Top cotton

Element 2 = 16 in (41 cm) = 6 strands of purple Double Top cotton

Element 3 = 16 in (41 cm) = 6 strands of pink Double Top cotton

Element 4 = 16 in (41 cm) = 6 strands of light pink Double Top cotton

Element 5 = 16 in (41 cm) = 6 strands of lilac Double Top cotton

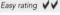

Method

Follow the method for Five-element, Two-ridge Braid (see page 80). Take care to keep all the strands together for each element.

FOUR COLORS 1:1:1:2

Easy rating ✔✔

Materials

Element 1 = 16 in (41 cm) = 6 strands of purple Double Top cotton

Element 2 = 16 in (41 cm) = 6 strands of lilac Double Top cotton

Element 3 = 16 in (41 cm) = 6 strands of light pink Double Top cotton

Element 4 = 16 in (41 cm) = 6 strands of pink Double Top cotton

Element 5 = 16 in (41 cm) = 6 strands of purple Double Top cotton

Method

Follow the method for Five-element, Two-ridge Braid (see page 80). Take care to keep all the strands together for each element.

FIVE COLORS

Easy rating ✔✔

Materials

Element 1 = 15 in (38 cm) = 10 strands of light gray No 5 pearl cotton

Element 2 = 15 in (38 cm) = 10 strands of gray No 5 pearl cotton

Element 3 = 15 in (38 cm) = 10 strands of dark gray No 5 pearl cotton

Element 4 = 15 in (38 cm) = 10 strands of pink No 5 pearl cotton

Element 5 = 15 in (38 cm) = 10 strands of light pink No 5 pearl cotton

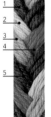

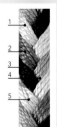

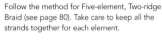

Method

Follow the method for Five-element, Two-ridge Braid (see page 80). Take care to keep all the strands together for each element.

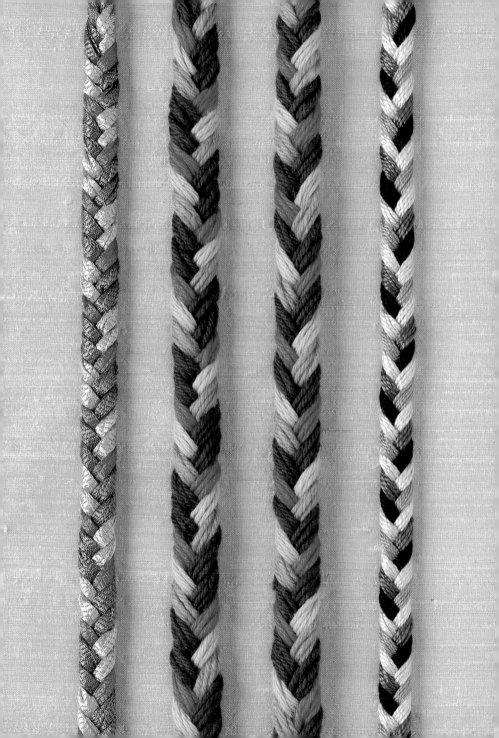

TWO TEXTURES
Easy rating ✔

Materials
Element 1 = 15 in (38 cm) = 1 strand of gray ruched knitting ribbon

Element 2 = 19 in (48 cm) = 1 strand of pink gimp

Element 3 = 19 in (48 cm) = 1 strand of pink gimp

Element 4 = 16 in (41 cm) = 1 strand of pink gimp

Element 5 = 15 in (38 cm) = 1 strand of gray ruched knitting ribbon

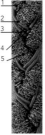

Method
Follow the method for Five-element, Two-ridge Braid (see page 80).

TWO TEXTURES
Easy rating ✔

Materials
Element 1 = 14 in (36 cm) = 1 strand of light pink rattail

Element 2 = 14 in (36 cm) = 1 strand of pink rattail

Element 3 = 14 in (36 cm) = 1 strand of light pink rattail

Element 4 = 14 in (36 cm) = 6 strands of gray Kid Classic wool

Element 5 = 14 in (36 cm) = 6 strands of gray Kid Classic wool

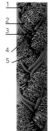

Method
Follow the method for Five-element, Two-ridge Braid (see page 80).

WITH BEADS
Easy rating ✔✔✔

Materials
Element 1 = 18 in (46 cm) = 1 strand of pink gimp, threaded with 17 4-mm gray glass beads

Element 2 = 18 in (46 cm) = 1 strand of pink gimp, threaded with 17 4-mm gray glass beads

Element 3 = 18 in (46 cm) = 1 strand of pink gimp, threaded with 17 4-mm gray glass beads

Element 4 = 18 in (46 cm) = 1 strand of pink gimp, threaded with 17 4-mm gray glass beads

Element 5 =18 in (45 cm) = 1 strand of pink gimp, threaded with 17 4-mm gray glass beads

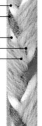

Method
Follow the method for Five-element, Two-ridge Braid (see page 80). The beads are added by pushing a bead up from the leftmost and rightmost elements. When they are resting against the outside edge of the work, work Steps 2 and 3, making sure that the beads remain on the outer edge of the braid. Work Steps 2 and 3 again (without beads), before repeating the whole process.

WITH BEADS
Easy rating ✔✔✔

Materials
Element 1 = 14 in (36 cm) = 1 string of gray size 11° rocaille beads

Element 2 = 14 in (36 cm) = 1 string of gray size 11° rocaille beads

Element 3 = 14 in (36 cm) = 1 string of gray size 11° rocaille beads

Element 4 = 14 in (36 cm) = 1 string of gray size 11° rocaille beads

Element 5 = 14 in (36 cm) = 1 string of gray size 11° rocaille beads

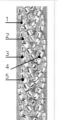

Method
Follow the method for Five-element, Two-ridge Braid (see page 80), taking care to keep the beads evenly spaced along the string.

Five-element, four-ridge braid

The odd number of elements make this a symmetrical braid. It is known by various names including French Sinnet, Five-end Mesh, Balanced Plain Interlacing, and Five-strand Flat Braid.

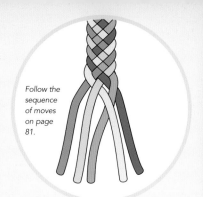

Follow the sequence of moves on page 81.

PLAIN

Easy rating ✔

Materials

Element 1 = 16 in (41 cm) = 1 strand of blue rattail

Element 2 = 16 in (41 cm) = 1 strand of blue rattail

Element 3 = 16 in (41 cm) = 1 strand of blue rattail

Element 4 = 16 in (41 cm) = 1 strand of blue rattail

Element 5 = 16 in (41 cm) = 1 strand of blue rattail

Method

Follow the method for Five-element, Four-ridge Braid (see page 81).

TWO COLORS 1:4

Easy rating ✔✔

Materials

Element 1 = 17 in (43 cm) = 8 strands of blue knitting ribbon
Element 2 = 17 in (43 cm) = 8 strands of pale blue knitting ribbon
Element 3 = 17 in (43 cm) = 8 strands of pale blue knitting ribbon
Element 4 = 17 in (43 cm) = 8 strands of pale blue knitting ribbon
Element 5 = 17 in (43 cm) = 8 strands of pale blue knitting ribbon

Method

Follow the method for Five-element, Four-ridge Braid (see page 81). Take care to keep all the strands together for each element.

TWO COLORS 2:3

Easy rating ✔✔

Materials

Element 1 = 15 in (38 cm) = 8 strands of green No 5 pearl cotton
Element 2 = 15 in (38 cm) = 8 strands of green No 5 pearl cotton
Element 3 = 15 in (38 cm) = 8 strands of pale green No 5 pearl cotton
Element 4 = 15 in (38 cm) = 8 strands of pale green No 5 pearl cotton
Element 5 = 15 in (38 cm) = 8 strands of pale green No 5 pearl cotton

Method

Follow the method for Five-element, Four-ridge Braid (see page 81). Take care to keep all the strands together for each element.

TWO COLORS 2:3

Easy rating ✔✔

Materials

Element 1 = 15 in (38 cm) = 8 strands of green No 5 pearl cotton
Element 2 = 15 in (38 cm) = 8 strands of pale green No 5 pearl cotton
Element 3 = 15 in (38 cm) = 8 strands of pale green No 5 pearl cotton
Element 4 = 15 in (38 cm) = 8 strands of pale green No 5 pearl cotton
Element 5 = 15 in (38 cm) = 8 strands of green No 5 pearl cotton

Method

Follow the method for Five-element, Four-ridge Braid (see page 81). Take care to keep all the strands together for each element.

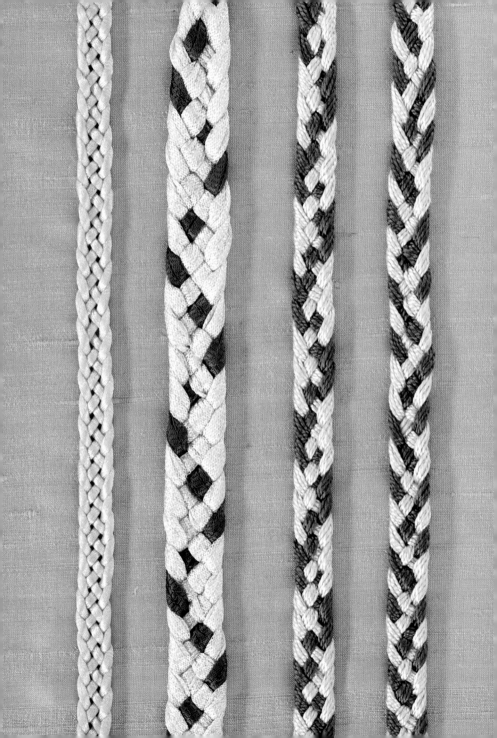

THREE COLORS 1:1:3

Easy rating ✔✔

Materials

Element 1 = 16 in (41 cm) = 6 strands of green No 5 pearl cotton

Element 2 = 16 in (41 cm) = 6 strands of blue No 5 pearl cotton

Element 3 = 16 in (41 cm) = 6 strands of pale green No 5 pearl cotton

Element 4 = 16 in (41 cm) = 6 strands of pale green No 5 pearl cotton

Element 5 = 16 in (41 cm) = 6 strands of pale green No 5 pearl cotton

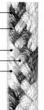

Method

Follow the method for Five-element, Four-ridge Braid (see page 81). Take care to keep all the strands together for each element

THREE COLORS 1:1:3

Easy rating ✔✔

Materials

Element 1 = 16 in (41 cm) = 6 strands of pale green No 5 pearl cotton

Element 2 = 16 in (41 cm) = 6 strands of green No 5 pearl cotton

Element 3 = 16 in (41 cm) = 6 strands of green No 5 pearl cotton

Element 4 = 16 in (41 cm) = 6 strands of green No 5 pearl cotton

Element 5 = 16 in (41 cm) = 6 strands of ocher No 5 pearl cotton

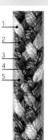

Method

Follow the method for Five-element, Four-ridge Braid (see page 81). Take care to keep all the strands together for each element.

THREE COLORS 1:2:2

Easy rating ✔✔

Materials

Element 1 = 17 in (43 cm) = 6 strands of pale green knitting ribbon

Element 2 = 17 in (43 cm) = 6 strands of ocher knitting ribbon

Element 3 = 17 in (43 cm) = 6 strands of green knitting ribbon

Element 4 = 17 in (43 cm) = 6 strands of green knitting ribbon

Element 5 = 17 in (43 cm) = 6 strands of pale green knitting ribbon

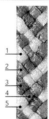

Method

Follow the method for Five-element, Four-ridge Braid (see page 81). Take care to keep all the strands together for each element.

THREE COLORS 1:2:2

Easy rating ✔✔

Materials

Element 1 = 17 in (43 cm) = 6 strands of blue knitting ribbon

Element 2 = 17 in (43 cm) = 6 strands of pale green knitting ribbon

Element 3 = 17 in (43 cm) = 6 strands of blue knitting ribbon

Element 4 = 17 in (43 cm) = 6 strands of green knitting ribbon

Element 5 = 17 in (43 cm) = 6 strands of green knitting ribbon

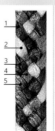

Method

Follow the method for Five-element, Four-ridge Braid (see page 81). Take care to keep all the strands together for each element.

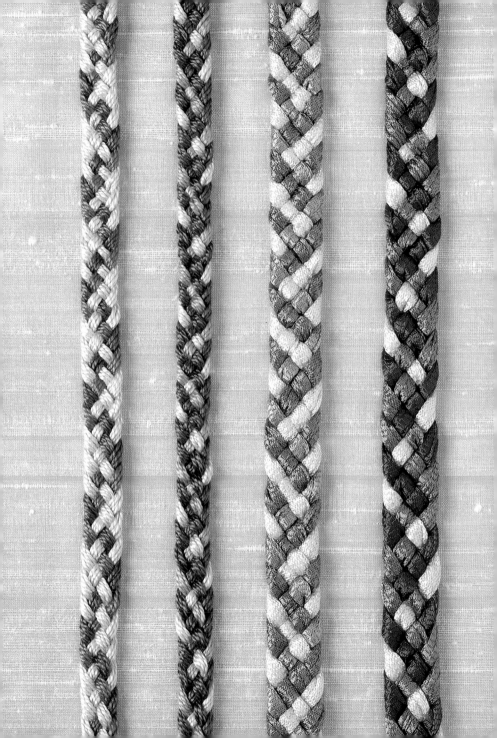

THREE COLORS 1:2:2

Materials

Element 1 = 17 in (43 cm) = 6 strands of ocher knitting ribbon

Element 2 = 17 in (43 cm) = 6 strands of green knitting ribbon

Element 3 = 17 in (43 cm) = 6 strands of green knitting ribbon

Element 4 = 17 in (43 cm) = 6 strands of pale green knitting ribbon

Element 5 = 17 in (43 cm) = 6 strands of pale green knitting ribbon

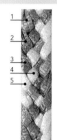

Method

Follow the method for Five-element, Four-ridge Braid (see page 81). Take care to keep all the strands together for each element.

FOUR COLORS 1:1:1:2

Materials

Element 1 = 17 in (43 cm) = 6 strands of green knitting ribbon

Element 2 = 17 in (43 cm) = 6 strands of green knitting ribbon

Element 3 = 17 in (43 cm) = 6 strands of light blue knitting ribbon

Element 4 = 17 in (43 cm) = 6 strands of dark blue knitting ribbon

Element 5 = 17 in (43 cm) = 6 strands of blue knitting ribbon

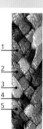
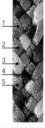

Method

Follow the method for Five-element, Four-ridge Braid (see page 81). Take care to keep all the strands together for each element.

FOUR COLORS 1:1:1:2

Materials

Element 1 = 17 in (43 cm) = 6 strands of blue knitting ribbon

Element 2 = 17 in (43 cm) = 6 strands of ocher knitting ribbon

Element 3 = 17 in (43 cm) = 6 strands of light blue knitting ribbon

Element 4 = 17 in (43 cm) = 6 strands of pale green knitting ribbon

Element 5 = 17 in (43 cm) = 6 strands of blue knitting ribbon

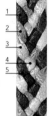

Method

Follow the method for Five-element, Four-ridge Braid (see page 81). Take care to keep all the strands together for each element.

FIVE COLORS

Materials

Element 1 = 17 in (43 cm) = 6 strands of blue knitting ribbon

Element 2 = 17 in (43 cm) = 6 strands of ocher knitting ribbon

Element 3 = 17 in (43 cm) = 6 strands of pale green knitting ribbon

Element 4 = 17 in (43 cm) = 6 strands of light blue knitting ribbon

Element 5 = 17 in (43 cm) = 6 strands of green knitting ribbon

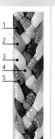

Method

Follow the method for Five-element, Four-ridge Braid (see page 81). Take care to keep all the strands together for each element.

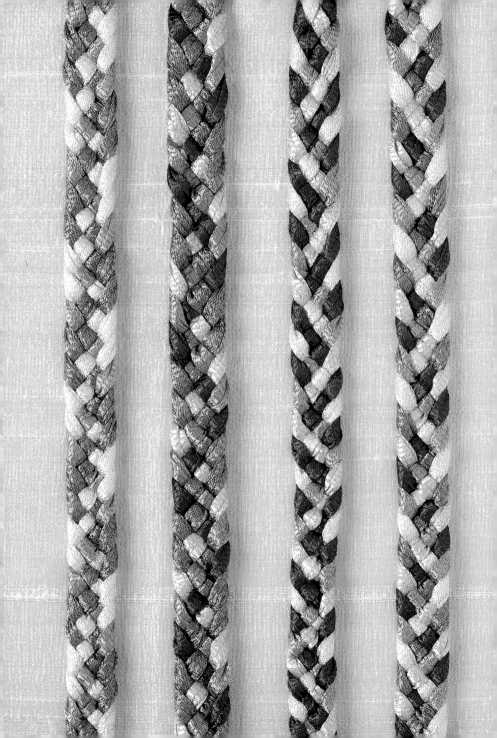

TWO TEXTURES
Easy rating ✔

Materials

Element 1 = 15 in (38 cm) = 1 strand of twisted green gimp cord

Element 2 = 15 in (38 cm) = 1 strand of pale green knitting ribbon

Element 3 = 15 in (38 cm) = 1 strand of pale green knitting ribbon

Element 4 = 15 in (38 cm) = 1 strand of pale green knitting ribbon

Element 5 = 15 in (38 cm) = 1 strand of pale green knitting ribbon

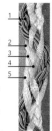

Method

Follow the method for Five-element, Four-ridge Braid (see page 81).

TWO TEXTURES
Easy rating ✔

Materials

Element 1 = 16 in (41 cm) = 6 strands of Summer Tweed

Element 2 = 16 in (41 cm) = 6 strands of Summer Tweed

Element 3 = 19 in (48 cm) = 1 strand of green gimp

Element 4 = 19 in (48 cm) = 1 strand of green gimp

Element 5 = 19 in (48 cm) = 1 strand of green gimp

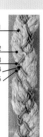

Method

Follow the method for Five-element, Four-ridge Braid (see page 81).

RIBBON
Easy rating ✔✔✔

Materials

Element 1 = 17 in (43 cm) = 1 strand of 10 mm blue ribbon

Element 2 = 17 in (43 cm) = 1 strand of 10 mm blue ribbon

Element 3 = 14 in (36 cm) = 1 strand of 3 mm pale green ribbon

Element 4 = 14 in (36 cm) = 1 strand of 3 mm pale green ribbon

Element 5 = 14 in (36 cm) = 1 strand of 3 mm pale green ribbon

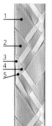

Method

Follow the method for Five-element, Four-ridge Braid (see page 81). Each ribbon will need to be folded at the edge of the braid. You may find it easier to work this sample on a corkboard so that you can pin down the edges. Iron the final braid to keep in the creases.

WITH BEADS
Easy rating ✔✔

Materials

Element 1 = 14 in (36 cm) = 1 string of green size 10° rocaille beads

Element 2 = 14 in (36 cm) = 1 string of green size 10° rocaille beads

Element 3 = 13 in (33 cm) = 1 strand of green Japanese braid

Element 4 = 13 in (33 cm) = 1 strand of green Japanese braid

Element 5 = 13 in (33 cm) = 1 strand of green Japanese braid

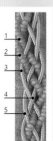

Method

Follow the method for Five-element, Four-ridge Braid (see page 81). Do not pull the elements too tight.

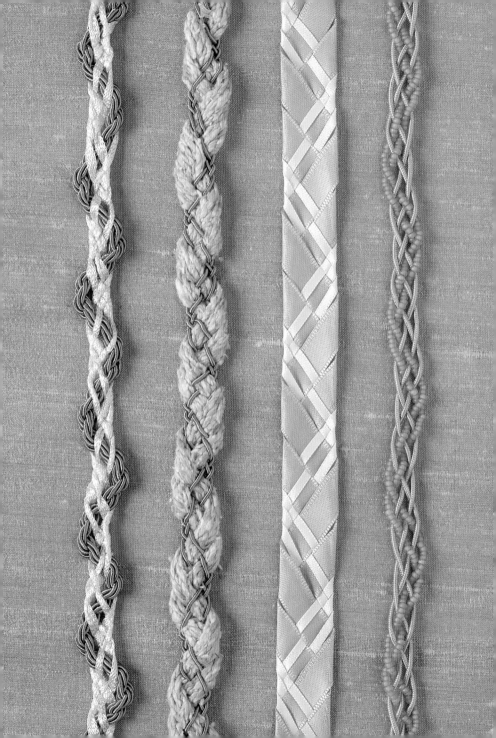

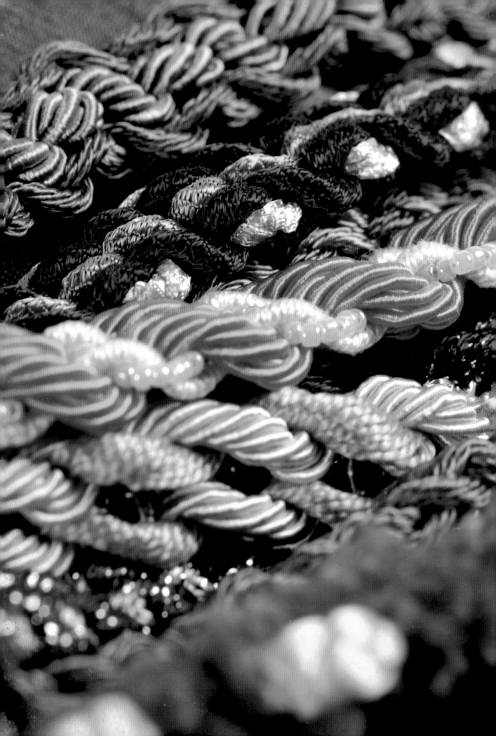

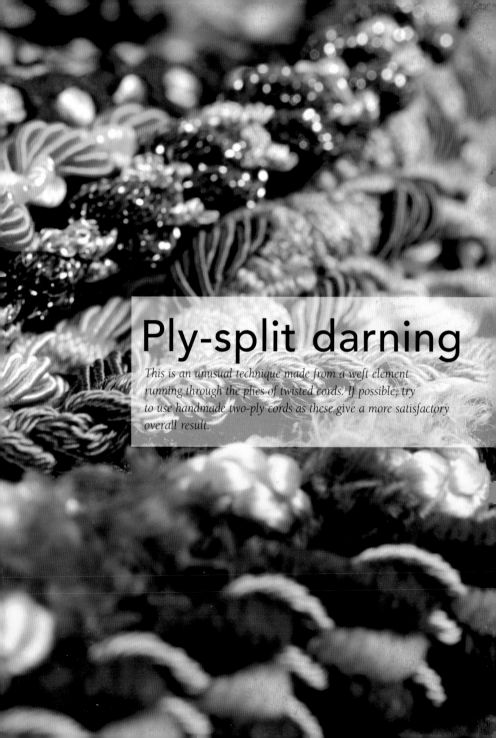

Ply-split darning

This is an unusual technique made from a weft element running through the plies of twisted cords. If possible, try to use handmade two-ply cords as these give a more satisfactory overall result.

Two Cords

Ply-split darning can be worked with any cord.
These samples are all made using two warp cords
and one weft element. The two-ply warps enable
the ply-splitting to be even, with one ply sitting
either side of the weft element. All the samples
are made with Z-twist cords.

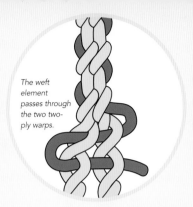

The weft element passes through the two two-ply warps.

PLAIN

Easy rating ✔

Materials

Element 1 = 19 in (48 cm) = 8 strands of yellow No 5
    pearl cotton
Element 2 = 14 in (36 cm) = 1 premade, plain yellow
    cord (ply 1 = 8 strands of yellow No 5 pearl cotton;
    ply 2 = 8 strands of yellow No 5 pearl cotton)
Element 3 = 14 in (36 cm) = 1 premade, plain yellow
    cord (ply 1 = 8 strands of yellow No 5 pearl cotton;
    ply 2 = 8 strands of yellow No 5 pearl cotton)

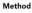
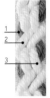

Method

Follow the instructions for Two Cord Ply-split
Darning (see page 84).

TWO COLORS

Easy rating ✔

Materials

Element 1 = 22 in (56 cm) = 4 strands of blue Double
    Top cotton
Element 2 = 15 in (38 cm) = 1 premade, plain yellow
    cord (ply 1 = 4 strands of yellow Double Top cotton;
    ply 2 = 4 strands of yellow Double Top cotton)
Element 3 = 15 in (38 cm) = 1 premade, plain yellow
    cord (ply 1 = 4 strands of yellow Double Top cotton;
    ply 2 = 4 strands of yellow Double Top cotton)

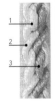

Method

Follow the instructions for Two Cord Ply-split
Darning (see page 84).

TWO COLORS

Easy rating ✔

Materials

Element 1 = 21 in (53 cm) = 6 strands of yellow
    knitting ribbon
Element 2 = 15 in (38 cm) = 1 premade, plain yellow
    cord (ply 1 = 6 strands of yellow knitting ribbon;
    ply 2 = 6 strands of yellow knitting ribbon)
Element 3 = 15 in (38 cm) = 1 premade, plain orange
    cord (ply 1 = 6 strands of orange knitting ribbon;
    ply 2 = 6 strands of orange knitting ribbon)

Method

Follow the instructions for Two Cord Ply-split
Darning (see page 84).

THREE COLORS

Easy rating ✔

Materials

Element 1 = 20 in (51 cm) = 4 strands of orange
    Double Top cotton
Element 2 = 14 in (36 cm) = 1 premade, plain navy
    cord (ply 1 = 4 strands of navy Double Top cotton;
    ply 2 = 4 strands of navy Double Top cotton)
Element 3 = 14 in (36 cm) = 1 premade, plain blue
    cord in length (ply 1 = 4 strands of blue Double Top
    cotton; ply 2 = 4 strands of blue Double Top cotton)

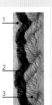

Method

Follow the instructions for Two Cord Ply-split
Darning (see page 84).

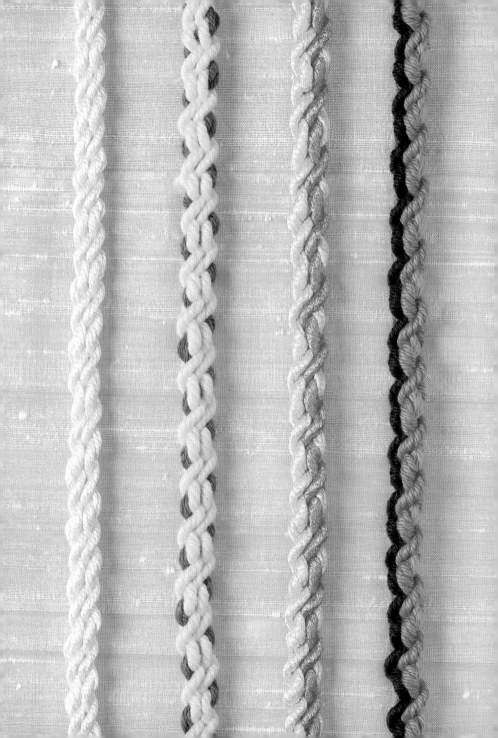

TWO COLORS, TWO-COLORED CORD

Materials

Element 1 = 20 in (51 cm) = 4 strands of yellow Double Top cotton

Element 2 = 14 in (36 cm) = 1 premade, two-colored cord (ply 1 = 4 strands of orange Double Top cotton; ply 2 = 4 strands of yellow Double Top cotton)

Element 3 = 14 in (36 cm) = 1 premade, plain yellow cord (ply 1 = 4 strands of yellow Double Top cotton; ply 2 = 4 strands of yellow Double Top cotton)

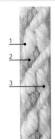

Method

Follow the instructions for Two Cord Ply-split Darning (see page 84). Make sure that the orange is the topmost ply for Step 2.

TWO COLORS, TWO-COLORED CORD

Materials

Element 1 = 21 in (53 cm) = 4 strands of yellow knitting ribbon

Element 2 =14 in (36 cm) = 1 premade, two-colored cord (ply 1 = 4 strands of blue knitting ribbon; ply 2 = 4 strands of yellow knitting ribbon)

Element 3 = 14 in (36 cm) = 1 premade, two-colored cord (ply 1 = 4 strands of blue knitting ribbon; ply 2 = 4 strands of yellow knitting ribbon)

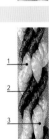

Method

Follow the instructions for Two Cord Ply-split Darning (see page 84). Make sure that the blue is the topmost ply for Steps 2 and 4.

TWO COLORS, TWO-COLORED CORD

Materials

Element 1 = 21 in (53 cm) = 4 strands of yellow knitting ribbon

Element 2 = 14 in (36 cm) = 1 premade, two-colored cord (ply 1 = 4 strands of blue knitting ribbon; ply 2 = 4 strands of yellow knitting ribbon)

Element 3 = 14 in (36 cm) = 1 premade, two-colored cord (ply 1 = 4 strands of blue knitting ribbon; ply 2 = 4 strands of yellow knitting ribbon)

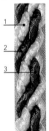

Method

Follow the instructions for Two Cord Ply-split Darning (see page 84). Make sure that the blue is the topmost ply for Step 2 and the yellow is topmost ply for Step 4.

THREE COLORS, TWO-COLORED CORD

Materials

Element 1 = 20 in (51 cm) = 4 strands of orange Double Top cotton

Element 2 = 14 in (36 cm) = 1 premade, two-colored cord (ply 1 = 4 strands of navy Double Top cotton; ply 2 = 4 strands of blue Double Top cotton)

Element 3 = 14 in (36 cm) = 1 premade, two-colored cord (ply 1 = 4 strands of navy Double Top cotton; ply 2 = 4 strands of blue Double Top cotton)

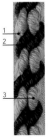

Method

Follow the instructions for Two Cord Ply-split Darning (see page 84). Make sure that the navy is the topmost ply when making Steps 2 and 4.

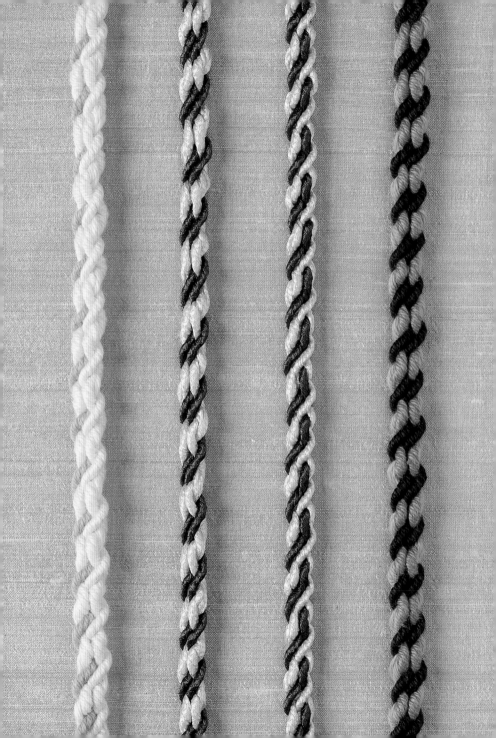

DIFFERENT THICKNESS

Easy rating ✓

Materials

Element 1 = 22 in (56 cm) = 4 strands of yellow Glitter viscose

Element 2 = 15 in (38 cm) = 1 premade, two-colored cord (ply 1 = 16 strands of blue Glitter viscose; ply 2 = 4 strands of yellow Glitter viscose)

Element 3 = 15 in (38 cm) = 1 premade, two-colored cord (ply 1 = 16 strands of blue Glitter viscose; ply 2 = 4 strands of yellow Glitter viscose)

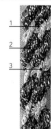

Method

Follow the instructions for Two Cord Ply-split Darning (see page 84). Make sure that the blue is the topmost when making Steps 2 and 4.

TWO TEXTURES

Easy rating ✓✓

Materials

Element 1 = 26 in (66 cm) = 1 strand of yellow crepe cord

Element 2 = 14 in (36 cm) = 1 premade, textured cord (ply 1 = 4 strands of blue Balmoral bouclé; ply 2 = 4 strands of blue Balmoral bouclé)

Element 3 = 14 in (36 cm) = 1 premade, textured cord (ply 1 = 4 strands of blue Balmoral bouclé; ply 2 = 4 strands of blue Balmoral bouclé)

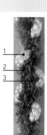

Method

Follow the instructions for Two Cord Ply-split Darning (see page 84). The textured yarn makes it difficult to find the space between the plies.

WITH BEADS

Easy rating ✓✓

Materials

Element 1 = 20 in (51 cm) = 1 strand of yellow gimp

Element 2 = 13 in (33 cm) = 1 premade, two-textured cord (ply 1 = 8 strands of yellow gimp; ply 2 = 16 strands of yellow No 5 pearl cotton)

Element 3 = 13 in (33 cm) = 1 premade, two-textured cord (ply 1 = 8 strands of yellow gimp; ply 2 = 16 strands of yellow No 5 pearl cotton)

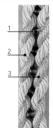

Method

Follow the instructions for Two Cord Ply-split Darning (see page 84), making sure that the gimp is the topmost ply in Steps 2 and 4. After Step 3, thread a bead onto Element 1 (the gimp weft) and push it up close to the work. Continue with the steps until you have completed Step 7. Thread another bead onto Element 1, before continuing to repeat the whole process.

WITH BEADS

Easy rating ✓✓

Materials

Element 1 = 20 in (51 cm) = 1 string of yellow size 11° rocaille beads

Element 2 = 13 in (33 cm) = 1 premade, textured cord (ply 1 = 8 strands of yellow No 5 pearl cotton; ply 2 = 8 strands of orange gimp)

Element 3 = 13 in (33 cm) =1 premade, textured cord (ply 1 = 8 strands of yellow No 5 pearl cotton; ply 2 = 8 strands of orange gimp)

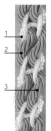

Method

Follow the instructions for Two Cord Ply-split Darning (see page 84), making sure that the gimp is the topmost ply in Steps 2 and 4.

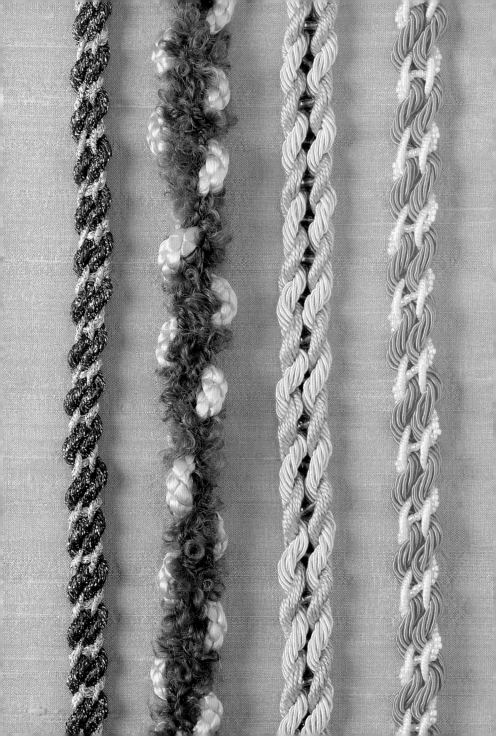

Three Cords

Working with more cords increases the width of the darning, as well as the pattern possibilities. Again, all samples are worked with Z-twist, two-ply cords.

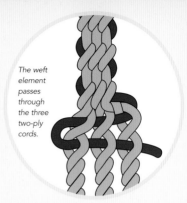

The weft element passes through the three two-ply cords.

PLAIN

Easy rating ✔

Materials

Element 1 = 25 in (64 cm) = 6 strands of cream Prism viscose
Element 2 = 14 in (36 cm) = 1 premade, plain cord (ply 1 = 6 strands of cream Prism viscose; ply 2 = 6 strands of cream Prism viscose)
Element 3 = 14 in (36 cm) = 1 premade, plain cord (ply 1 = 6 strands of cream Prism viscose; ply 2 = 6 strands of cream Prism viscose)
Element 4 = 14 in (36 cm) = 1 premade, plain cord (ply 1 = 6 strands of cream Prism viscose; ply 2 = 6 strands of cream Prism viscose)

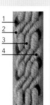

Method

Follow the instructions for Three Cord Ply-split Darning (see page 86).

TWO COLORS

Easy rating ✔

Materials

Element 1 = 26 in (66 cm) = 4 strands of purple Chunky wool
Element 2 = 13 in (33 cm) = 1 premade, plain mauve cord (ply 1 = 4 strands of mauve Chunky wool; ply 2 = 4 strands of mauve Chunky wool)
Element 3 = 13 in (33 cm) = 1 premade, plain mauve cord (ply 1 = 4 strands of mauve Chunky wool; ply 2 = 4 strands of mauve Chunky wool)
Element 4 = 13 in (33 cm) = 1 premade, plain mauve cord (ply 1 = 4 strands of mauve Chunky wool; ply 2 = 4 strands of mauve Chunky wool)

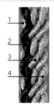

Method

Follow the instructions for Three Cord Ply-split Darning (see page 86).

TWO COLORS

Easy rating ✔

Materials

Element 1 = 27 in (69 cm) = 6 strands of mauve knitting ribbon
Element 2 = 14 in (36 cm) = 1 premade, burgundy cord (ply 1 = 6 strands of burgundy knitting ribbon; ply 2 = 6 strands of burgundy knitting ribbon)
Element 3 = 14 in (36 cm) = 1 premade, mauve cord (ply 1 = 6 strands of mauve knitting ribbon; ply 2 = 6 strands of mauve knitting ribbon)
Element 4 = 14 in (36 cm) = 1 premade, mauve cord (ply 1 = 6 strands of mauve knitting ribbon; ply 2 = 6 strands of mauve knitting ribbon)

Method

Follow the instructions for Three Cord Ply-split Darning (see page 86).

TWO COLORS

Easy rating ✔

Materials

Element 1 = 25 in (64 cm) = 6 strands of ocher Prism viscose
Element 2 = 14 in (36 cm) = 1 premade, ocher cord (ply 1 = 6 strands of ocher Prism viscose; ply 2 = 6 strands of ocher Prism viscose)
Element 3 = 14 in (36 cm) = 1 premade, mauve cord (ply 1 = 6 strands of mauve Prism viscose; ply 2 = 6 strands of mauve Prism viscose)
Element 4 = 14 in (36 cm) = 1 premade, ocher cord (ply 1 = 6 strands of ocher Prism viscose; ply 2 = 6 strands of ocher Prism viscose)

Method

Follow the instructions for Three Cord Ply-split Darning (see page 86).

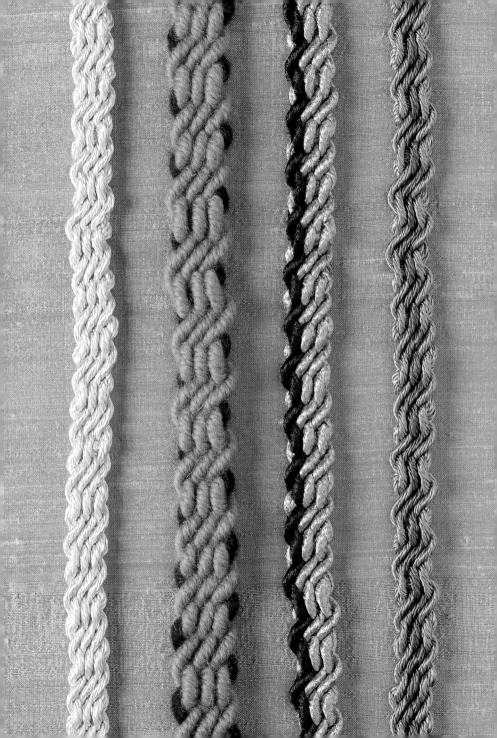

TWO COLORS

Easy rating ✔

Materials

Element 1 = 25 in (64 cm) = 6 strands of burgundy
Prism viscose

Element 2 = 14 in (36 cm) = 1 premade, mauve cord
(ply 1 = 6 strands of mauve Prism viscose; ply 2 =
6 strands of mauve Prism viscose)

Element 3 = 14 in (36 cm) = 1 premade, burgundy
cord (ply 1 = 6 strands of burgundy Prism viscose;
ply 2 = 6 strands of burgundy Prism viscose)

Element 4 = 14 in (36 cm) = 1 premade, mauve cord
(ply 1 = 6 strands of mauve Prism viscose; ply 2 =
6 strands of mauve Prism viscose)

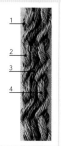

Method

Follow the instructions for Three Cord Ply-
split Darning (see page 86).

FOUR COLORS

Easy rating ✔

Materials

Element 1 = 27 in (69 cm) = 6 strands of cream
knitting ribbon

Element 2 = 14 in (36 cm) = 1 premade, burgundy
cord (ply 1 = 6 strands of burgundy knitting ribbon;
ply 2 = 6 strands of burgundy knitting ribbon)

Element 3 = 14 in (36 cm) = 1 premade, ocher cord
(ply 1 = 6 strands of ocher knitting ribbon; ply 2 =
6 strands of ocher knitting ribbon)

Element 4 = 14 in (36 cm) = 1 premade, purple cord
(ply 1 = 6 strands of purple knitting ribbon; ply 2 =
6 strands of purple knitting ribbon)

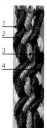

Method

Follow the instructions for Three Cord Ply-
split Darning (see page 86).

TWO COLORS, TWO-COLORED CORD

Easy rating ✔

Materials

Element 1 = 27 in (69 cm) = 6 strands of purple
knitting ribbon

Element 2 = 14 in (36 cm) = 1 premade, two-colored
cord (ply 1 = 6 strands of purple knitting ribbon;
ply 2 = 6 strands of ocher knitting ribbon)

Element 3 = 14 in (36 cm) = 1 premade, purple cord
(ply 1 = 6 strands of purple knitting ribbon; ply 2 =
6 strands of purple knitting ribbon)

Element 4 = 14 in (36 cm) = 1 premade, purple cord
(ply 1 = 6 strands of purple knitting ribbon; ply 2 =
6 strands of purple knitting ribbon)

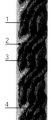

Method

Follow the instructions for Three Cord Ply-split
Darning (see page 86), making sure that the purple
is the topmost ply in Step 2.

TWO COLORS, TWO-COLORED CORD

Easy rating ✔

Materials

Element 1 = 25 in (64 cm) = 6 strands of mauve Prism
viscose

Element 2 = 14 in (36 cm) = 1 premade, mauve cord
(ply 1 = 6 strands of mauve Prism viscose; ply 2 = 6
strands of mauve Prism viscose)

Element 3 = 14 in (36 cm) = 1 premade, two-colored
cord (ply 1 = 6 strands of ocher Prism viscose; ply 2
= 6 strands of mauve Prism viscose)

Element 4 = 14 in (36 cm) = 1 premade, mauve cord
(ply 1 = 6 strands of mauve Prism viscose; ply 2 = 6
strands of mauve Prism viscose)

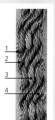

Method

Follow the instructions for Three Cord Ply-split
Darning (see page 86), making sure that the ocher
is the topmost ply in Step 3.

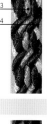

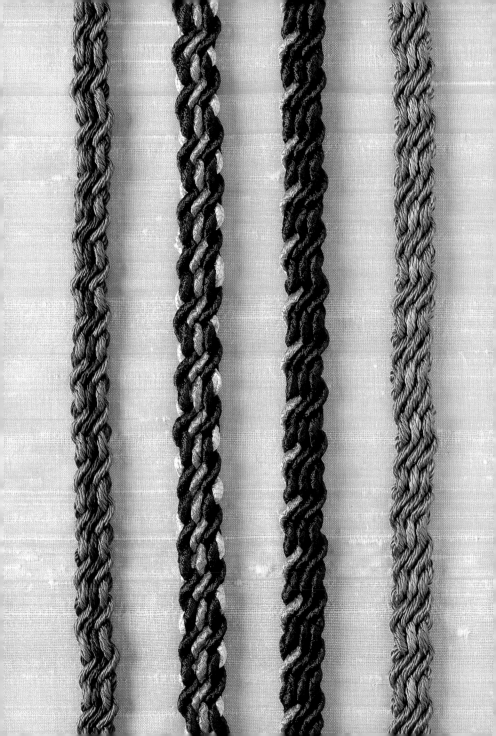

TWO COLORS, TWO-COLORED CORD

Materials

Element 1 = 26 in (66 cm) = 4 strands of purple
Chunky wool

Element 2 = 13 in (33 cm) = 1 premade, two-colored
cord (ply 1 = 4 strands of mauve Chunky wool; ply
2 = 4 strands of purple Chunky wool)

Element 3 = 13 in (33 cm) = 1 premade, plain purple
cord (ply 1 = 4 strands of purple Chunky wool; ply
2 = 4 strands of purple Chunky wool)

Element 4 = 13 in (33 cm) = 1 premade, two-colored
cord (ply 1 = 4 strands of mauve Chunky wool; ply
2 = 4 strands of purple Chunky wool)

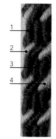

Method

Follow the instructions for Three Cord Ply-split
Darning (see page 86), making sure that the purple is
the topmost ply in Steps 2, 3, and 4.

TWO COLORS, TWO-COLORED CORD

Materials

Element 1 = 25 in (64 cm) = 6 strands of burgundy
Prism viscose

Element 2 = 14 in (36 cm) = 1 premade, two-colored
cord (ply 1 = 6 strands of ocher Prism viscose; ply 2
= 6 strands of burgundy Prism viscose)

Element 3 = 14 in (36 cm) = 1 premade, two-colored
cord (ply 1 = 6 strands of ocher Prism viscose; ply 2
= 6 strands of burgundy Prism viscose)

Element 4 = 14 in (36 cm) = 1 premade, burgundy
cord (ply 1 = 6 strands of burgundy Prism viscose;
ply 2 = 6 strands of burgundy Prism viscose)

Method

Follow the instructions for Three Cord Ply-split
Darning (see page 86), making sure that the ocher is
the topmost ply in Steps 2 and 3.

TWO COLORS, TWO-COLORED CORD

Materials

Element 1 = 25 in (64 cm) = 6 strands of mauve Prism
viscose

Element 2 = 14 in (36 cm) = 1 premade, two-colored
cord (ply 1 = 6 strands of ocher Prism viscose; ply 2
= 6 strands of mauve Prism viscose)

Element 3 = 14 in (36 cm) = 1 premade, two-colored
cord (ply 1 = 6 strands of ocher Prism viscose; ply 2
= 6 strands of mauve Prism viscose)

Element 4 = 14 in (36 cm) = 1 premade, two-colored
cord (ply 1 = 6 strands of ocher Prism viscose; ply 2
= 6 strands of mauve Prism viscose)

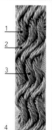

Method

Follow the instructions for Three Cord Ply-split
Darning (see page 86), making sure that the mauve
is the topmost ply in Steps 2, 3, and 4.

TWO COLORS, TWO-COLORED CORD

Materials

Element 1 = 25 in (64 cm) = 6 strands of mauve Prism
viscose

Element 2 = 14 in (36 cm) = 1 premade, two-colored
cord (ply 1 = 6 strands of ocher Prism viscose; ply 2
= 6 strands of mauve Prism viscose)

Element 3 = 14 in (36 cm) = 1 premade, two-colored
cord (ply 1 = 6 strands of ocher Prism viscose; ply 2
= 6 strands of mauve Prism viscose)

Element 4 = 14 in (36 cm) = 1 premade, two-colored
cord (ply 1 = 6 strands of ocher Prism viscose; ply 2
= 6 strands of mauve Prism viscose)

Method

Follow the instructions for Three Cord Ply-split Darning
(see page 86), making sure that the mauve is the
topmost ply in Steps 2 and 4. The ocher needs to be
the topmost ply in Step 3.

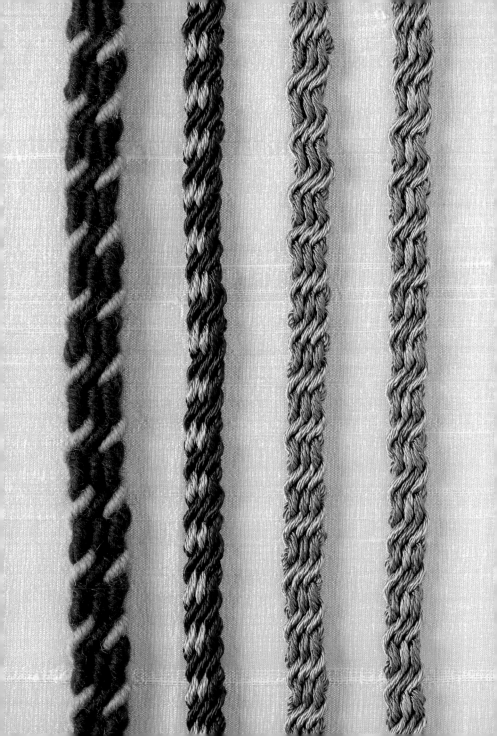

TWO TEXTURES

Materials

Element 1 = 24 in (61 cm) = 6 strands of mauve Prism viscose

Element 2 = 13 in (33 cm) 1 premade, mauve cord (ply 1 = 6 strands of mauve Prism viscose; ply 2 = 6 strands of mauve Prism viscose)

Element 3 = 13 in (33 cm) = 1 premade, ocher cord (ply 1 = 6 strands of ocher gimp; ply 2 = 6 strands of ocher gimp)

Element 4 = 13 in (33 cm) = 1 premade, mauve cord (ply 1 = 6 strands of mauve Prism viscose; ply 2 = 6 strands of mauve Prism viscose)

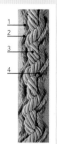

Method

Follow the instructions for Three Cord Ply-split Darning (see page 86).

TWO TEXTURES

Materials

Element 1 = 23 in (58 cm) = 2 strands of purple Chunky wool

Element 2 = 13 in (33 cm) = 1 premade, two-textured cord (ply 1 = 6 strands of ocher Prism viscose; ply 2 = 6 strands of purple Chunky wool)

Element 3 = 13 in (33 cm) = 1 premade, two-textured cord (ply 1 = 6 strands of ocher Prism viscose; ply 2 = 6 strands of mauve Chunky wool)

Element 4 = 13 in (33 cm) = 1 premade, two-textured cord (ply 1 = 6 strands of ocher Prism viscose; ply 2 = 6 strands of purple Chunky wool)

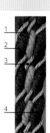

Method

Follow the instructions for Three Cord Ply-split Darning (see page 86), making sure that the wool is the topmost ply in Steps 2, 3, and 4.

TWO TEXTURES

Materials

Element 1 = 24 in (61 cm) = 2 strands of purple Chunky wool

Element 2 = 13 in (33 cm) = 1 premade, purple cord (ply 1 = 4 strands of purple Chunky wool; ply 2 = 4 strands of purple Chunky wool)

Element 3 = 13 in (33 cm) = 1 premade, two-textured cord (ply 1 = 1 strand of ocher ruched knitting ribbon; ply 2 = 4 strands of purple Chunky wool)

Element 4 = 13 in (33 cm) = 1 premade, purple cord (ply 1 = 4 strands of purple Chunky wool; ply 2 = 4 strands of purple Chunky wool)

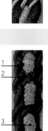

Method

Follow the instructions for Three Cord Ply-split Darning (see page 86), making sure that the ruched ribbon is the topmost ply in Step 3.

THREE TEXTURES

Materials

Element 1 = 22 in (56 cm) = 1 premade cord (ply 1 = 10 strands of ocher No 5 pearl cotton; ply 2 = 10 strands of ocher No 5 pearl cotton)

Element 2 = 13 in (33 cm) = 1 premade, two-textured cord (ply 1 = 10 strands of ocher No 5 pearl cotton; ply 2 = 8 strands of mauve gimp)

Element 3 = 13 in (33 cm) = 1 premade, two-textured cord (ply 1 = 10 strands of ocher No 5 pearl cotton; ply 2 = 1 strand of mauve ruched knitting ribbon)

Element 4 = 13 in (33 cm) = 1 premade, two-textured cord (ply 1 = 10 strands of ocher No 5 pearl cotton; ply 2 = 8 strands of mauve gimp)

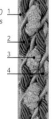

Method

Follow the instructions for Three Cord Ply-split Darning (see page 86), making sure that the gimp is the topmost ply in Steps 2 and 4. Keep the ocher pearl cotton the topmost ply in Step 3.

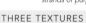

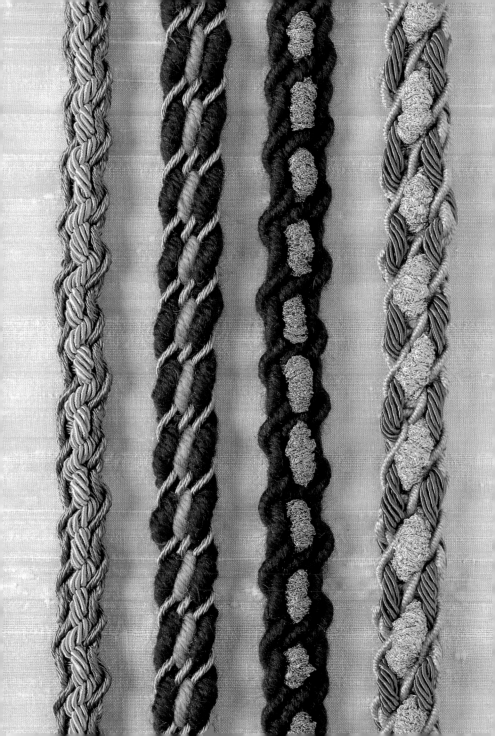

Resources

Pearl cotton thread
DMC threads
S. Hackensack Ave
Port Kearny Bldg 10F
South Kearny NJ 07032
(973) 589–0606
www.dmc-usa.com

Cotton and calmer cotton yarns
Rowan distributed by Westminster Fibers
4 Townsend West, #8
Nashua NH 03063
(603) 886–5054
www.westminsterfibers.com

Wool and synthetic yarns
Halcyon Yarn
12 School St.
Bath ME 04530
(207) 442–7909
www.halcyonyarn.com

Braiding equipment and Japanese silk braid
Carey Company
Summercourt, Ridgeway
Ottery St Mary
Devon, EX11 1DT
UK
+44 (0)1404 813–486
www.careycompany.com

Knitting ribbon, cord, and braid
Kreinik Mfg. Co.
1708 Gihon Rd
Parkersburg WV 26102
(304) 422–7178
www.lacis.com

Gimp, soutache (Russia braid), and rattail
Lacis
3163 Adeline St.
Berkeley CA 94703
(510) 843–2641
www.lacis.com

Silk ribbon
The Thread Gatherer
2108 Norcrest Dr.
Boise ID 83705
(208) 387–2641
www.threadgatherer.com

Beads
Mill Hill
N162 Hwy 35
Stoddard WI 54658
(608) 788–4600
www.millhillbeads.com

Index

Page numbers in *italics* refer to captions

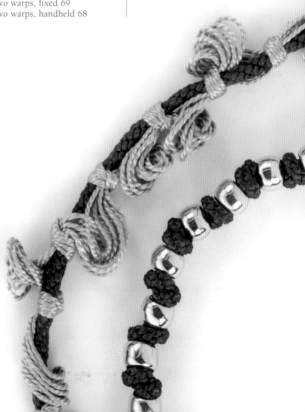

Credits

Author Acknowledgments

Thanks to my supportive family and the team at Quarto.

Quarto would like to thank and acknowledge the following for generously supplying yarns, beads, and silks used in the book:

Texere Yarns
+44 (0)1274 722 191
www.texere.co.uk

Rowan
+44 (0)1484 681 881
www.knitrowan.com

Beadworks
+44 (0)208 8553 3240
www.beadworks.co.uk

Henry Bertrand
+44 (0)207 349 1477
www.henrybertrand.co.uk

Picture Credits

Quarto would also like to thank and acknowledge the following for supplying photographs reproduced in this book:

Key: l = left, r = right
p6, p7 V&A Images/Victoria and Albert Museum
p66r Schacht Spindle Co. Inc. www.schachtspindle.com
p72l Carrow House; The Costume and Textile Study Centre; Norfolk Museums & Archaeology Service www.museums.norfolk.gov.uk